_____ 님께

_____ 드림

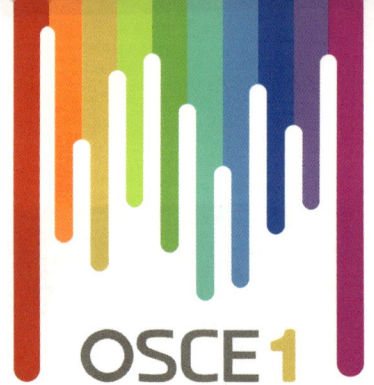

국제간호사를 위한 임상술기시험

첫째판 1쇄 인쇄 | 2025년 4월 5일
　　　　1쇄 발행 | 2025년 4월 10일

저　　　자 | 김라경
발　행　인 | 모형중
편　집　인 | 모형중
디　자　인 | 이명호

발　행　처 | 포널스
등　　　록 | 제2017-000021호
본　　　사 | 서울시 강북구 노해로8길22 경남아너스 3층
창　　　고 | 서울시 강북구 노해로8길22 경남아너스 2층
전　　　화 | 02-905-9671　　Fax | 02-905-9670

ⓒFORNURSE 2025년, 국제간호사를 위한 임상술기시험 OSCE Vol.1
Copyright©2025 ALL RIGHTS RESERVED

본서는 지은이와의 계약에 의해 포널스 출판사에서 발행합니다.
본서의 내용 및 삽화 일부 혹은 전부를 무단으로 전재 및 복제하는 것은 법으로 엄격히 금지되어 있습니다.

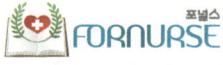
www.fornursebook.com

📖 도서 반품과 파본 교환은 본사로 문의하시기 바랍니다.
📖 검인은 저자와의 합의로 생략합니다.

ISBN 979-11-6627-640-8　　93510
정　가 25,000원

국제간호사를 위한
임상술기시험
OSCE VOLUME 1

Objective Structured Clinical Examinations
객관적 구조와 임상 시험

김라경 지음

FORNURSE

Prologue

사람마다 추구하는 꿈이 다르고 목표가 다르기 때문에, 각자의 인생 경로는 다양하고 독특합니다. 어떤 사람은 학문적 성취를 꿈꾸며 연구와 공부에 몰두하고, 또 어떤 사람은 창의적인 예술 활동을 통해 자신의 열정을 표현합니다. 또한, 누군가는 안정적인 직업과 가족을 이루는 것을 목표로 하기도 합니다. 이와 같은 개인의 다양한 목표와 꿈은 삶의 다양성을 보여주며, 우리의 사회를 더욱 풍요롭게 만듭니다.

인생의 여정에서 새로운 도전을 시작하는 것은 때로는 두렵지만, 그만큼 가치 있는 일입니다. 특히 간호사라는 전문직을 가지고 새로운 나라에서 경력을 이어가고자 하는 결정은 큰 용기가 필요한 선택일 것입니다.

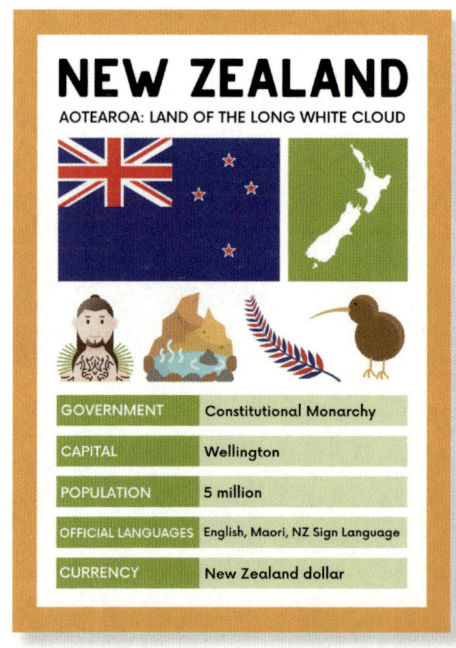

뉴질랜드는 깨끗한 자연환경과 높은 삶의 질, 그리고 전문직 종사자들을 위한 우수한 근무 환경으로 전 세계의 주목을 받고 있습니다. 특히 의료 분야에서는 체계적인 시스템과 전문성을 인정받는 환경이 마련되어 있어, 많은 한국 간호사들이 새로운 기회를 찾아 뉴질랜드로의 진출을 고려하고 있습니다.

To become a Nurse in New Zealand 전자책을 발간하고 뉴질랜드 간호사를 꿈꾸는 많은 선생님들과 1:1 강의를 진행한 지 2년이 되어갑니다. 이 과정에서 저는 다양한 경력과 열정을 가진 분들을 만나며 함께 성장할 수 있었습니다. 확신할 수 있는 것은, 뉴질랜드 간호사라는 목표는 분명 도달 가능한 꿈이라는 것입니다.

2024년 말부터 뉴질랜드 간호협회(Nursing Council of New Zealand, NCNZ)는 해외 간호사 등록 절차에 새로운 변화를 도입했습니다. 이 변경 사항은 국제적으로 자격을 갖춘 간호사(Internationally qualified nurses : IQN)들이 뉴질랜드에서 일하기 위한 절차를 단순화하고 보다 공정하고 일관된 평가를 제공하는 것을 목표로 합니다. 변경 사항에 대한 자세한 정보는 뉴질랜드 간호협회 웹사이트에서 확인할 수 있습니다.

김 라 경

Part I

1장 해외 간호사가 되기 위한 OSCE란 무엇인가?   9

임상술기란 무엇인가?　　　　　　　　　　　　　　　10

임상술기의 목적　　　　　　　　　　　　　　　　　11

뉴질랜드 간호협회 OSCE의 구성　　　　　　　　　　12

OSCE 준비 방법　　　　　　　　　　　　　　　　　13

OSCE의 평가기준　　　　　　　　　　　　　　　　14

2장은 무지개 색상으로 구분하여 OSCE 시험의 특징적인 10가지 스테이션을 부각시키고, 각 영역별의 독특한 특성을 강조하고자 합니다.

3장에서는 10개 스테이션별로 1개의 세부적인 시나리오를 담아, 보다 깊이 있는 이해를 돕고자 합니다.

Part II

2장 핵심 간호술기와 10단계 수행절차, 체크리스트   19

NZNC OSCE Scenarios   20

❶ 정신 건강 사정
Mental Health Assessment   22

❷ 신체사정(활력징후 측정)
Physiological assessment   33

❸ 세부 생리학적 사정
Specific physiological assessment   47

❹ 전문적인 답변
Professional Responsibility   57

❺ 응급상황 관리
Emergency management   79

❻ 임상 술기(상처드레싱 교환)
Clinical skills   95

❼ 약물 투약
Medication Administration   109

❽ 의사소통 및 팀워크
Communication and teamwork   123

❾ 간호계획 수립
Planning nursing care   135

❿ 위급한 상태의 환자 관리
Managing the deteriorating patient   149

Contents

3장 10단계 예문과 단계별 1개 연습 시나리오 167

❶ 정신 건강 사정 168
연습 Scenario 1: Excessive anxiety and worry 178

❷ 신체사정(활력징후 측정) 183
연습 Scenario 1: Chest pain 191

❸ 세부 생리학적 사정 197
연습 Scenario 1: Vaginal Packing removal for Patient with ongoing Bleeding 207

❹ 전문적인 답변 215
연습 Scenario 1: Handling Confidential Information 222

❺ 응급상황 관리 227
연습 Scenario 1: Cardiac Arrest 236

❻ 임상 술기(상처드레싱 교환) 243
연습 Scenario 1: Performing ECG 253

❼ 약물 투약 259
연습 Scenario 1: Intravenous medication administration 264

❽ 의사소통 및 팀워크 269
연습 Scenario 1: Interdisciplinary Team Meeting. 274

❾ 간호계획 수립 279
연습 Scenario 1: Chronic Disease Management 285

❿ 위급한 상태의 환자 관리 291
연습 Scenario 1: Acute Stroke 298

Part I

1장

해외 간호사가 되기 위한 OSCE란 무엇인가?

해외에서 간호사로 일하기 위해서는 각 나라별로 요구되는 자격 요건을 충족해야 합니다. 그 중 하나가 바로 OSCE(객관적 구조화 임상 시험)입니다. OSCE는 간호사의 임상 능력과 의사소통 능력을 평가하기 위한 시험입니다. 특히 영국이나 호주와 같은 국가에서는 해외 간호사들이 필수적으로 통과해야 하는 시험으로 자리 잡고 있습니다.

OSCE가 무엇인지, 준비 방법, 그리고 시험의 구성 요소에 대해 자세히 알아보겠습니다.

임상술기란 무엇인가?

OSCE(Objective Structured Clinical Examinations)는 시뮬레이션 환자와 상호 작용을 통해 간호사의 실무 능력을 평가하는 시험입니다. 시험은 다양한 상황에서의 간호 기술과 의사소통 능력을 평가하기 위해 여러 개의 '스테이션'으로 구성됩니다. 각 스테이션에서 간호사는 특정 임상 시나리오를 해결해야 하며, 평가자는 이를 바탕으로 점수를 매깁니다.

임상술기의 목적

OSCE는 간호사가 실제 임상 환경에서 환자를 적절히 돌볼 수 있는지를 평가하기 위해 고안되었습니다. 이는 단순히 이론적 지식만을 평가하는 것이 아니라, 실제 상황에서의 문제 해결 능력, 비판적 사고, 의사소통 능력, 그리고 기술적 능력을 모두 포함합니다. 따라서 간호사로서의 전반적인 역량을 종합적으로 검증할 수 있습니다.

뉴질랜드 간호협회 OSCE의 구성

뉴질랜드 간호협회(NCNZ)의 OSCE는 10개의 스테이션으로 구성되며, 각 스테이션에서 간호사는 다양한 임상 시나리오를 다루게 됩니다. 예를 들어, 환자 평가, 약물 관리, 응급 상황 대처, 상처 관리, 그리고 환자 교육 등이 포함될 수 있습니다. 각 스테이션은 약 12분 정도 소요되며, 간호사는 주어진 시간 내에 해당 시나리오를 해결해야 합니다.

2분 시나리오 읽기 → 8분 시나리오 해결 → 2분 다음 스테이션 이동

OSCE 준비 방법

기본 간호 지식 숙지: OSCE는 임상 상황을 다루기 때문에 기본적인 간호 지식이 매우 중요합니다. 이를 위해 교과서나 간호학 관련 서적을 통해 기초 지식을 충분히 숙지해야 합니다.

- **실습 경험 쌓기:** 실제 임상 경험은 OSCE 준비에 큰 도움이 됩니다. 가능한 한 많은 실습 기회를 통해 다양한 상황에 대한 대처 능력을 길러야 합니다.

- **모의 시험 참여:** OSCE 모의시험을 통해 형식에 익숙해지고, 실전 감각을 기를 수 있습니다.

- **피드백 수용:** 모의 시험 후에는 평가자로부터 피드백을 받아야 합니다. 이를 통해 자신의 약점을 보완하고, 실력을 향상시킬 수 있습니다.

- **동료와의 연습:** 동료 간호사와 함께 연습하는 것도 좋은 방법입니다. 서로의 피드백을 통해 부족한 부분을 개선할 수 있습니다.

OSCE의 평가기준

뉴질랜드 간호사 OSCE 평가 기준은 간호사가 실무에서 환자에게 안전하고 효과적인 간호를 제공할 수 있는지를 평가하는 데 중점을 둡니다.

안전성(Safety)

환자와 간호사의 안전은 간호 실무의 기본입니다. OSCE에서 안전성은 다음과 같은 기준으로 평가됩니다.

환자 안전:
- 절차를 시행하기 전에 반드시 환자의 신원을 확인했는가?
- 침대 난간을 올리는 등 환자의 낙상 예방 조치를 취했는가?
- 침습적 절차(예: 주사, 채혈 등)를 시행할 때 감염 예방 지침(손 위생, 장갑 착용 등)을 준수했는가?
- 약물을 투여하기 전, 약물의 이름, 용량, 그리고 환자의 알레르기 유무를 확인했는가?

↳ 자기 안전:
- 개인 보호 장비(PPE)를 올바르게 착용했는가?
- 감염성 폐기물을 적절히 처리했는가?
- 작업 환경에서 위험 요소(예: 물이 흐른 바닥, 날카로운 물체 등)를 인지하고 대응했는가?

효과성(Effectiveness)

간호 중재가 환자에게 긍정적인 영향을 미치는지를 평가합니다. 이 기준은 간호사가 임상적 판단을 기반으로 올바른 중재를 선택하고 이를 성공적으로 수행하는지를 보는 데 초점을 둡니다. 효과성을 높이기 위해 간호사는 근거 기반 간호(Evidence-Based Practice)를 바탕으로 실무를 수행해야 합니다.

↳ 중재의 적절성:
- 환자의 상태를 철저히 사정한 후, 그에 적합한 간호 중재를 선택했는가?
- 절차를 시행할 때 간호 표준과 지침을 따랐는가?

↳ 중재 결과:
- 중재가 환자의 상태를 개선하거나 문제를 완화했는가?(예: 통증 감소, 혈압 안정화 등)
- 환자의 반응을 관찰하고, 필요시 계획을 조정했는가?

🔖 전문성(Professionalism)

전문성은 간호사의 태도, 행동, 그리고 윤리적 실천을 포함합니다. OSCE에서는 간호사가 전문적인 태도를 유지하는지 평가합니다. 전문성은 간호사가 환자에게 신뢰를 주고, 동료 의료진과 협력할 수 있는 능력을 보여줍니다.

⤳ **윤리적 행동:**
- 환자의 프라이버시를 존중하고, 민감한 정보를 보호했는가?
- 환자의 동의를 구한 후 절차를 수행했는가?

⤳ **전문적 태도:**
- 환자에게 존중과 공감을 표현했는가?
- 차분하고 침착한 태도로 환자와 상호작용했는가?

⤳ **책임감:**
- 자신의 한계를 인식하고, 필요시 적절한 도움을 요청했는가?
- 지침을 따르고, 간호사로서의 책임을 다했는가?

🔖 의사소통 능력(Communication Skills)

OSCE에서 의사소통 능력은 환자와 의료진과의 명확하고 효과적인 상호작용을 평가합니다. 이는 간호사가 환자 중심의 간호를 제공할 수 있는지를 보여주는 핵심 요소입니다. 의사소통 능력은 간호사가 환자와 의료진 사이에서 중요한 중재자 역할을 수행할 수 있는지를 보여줍니다.

↳ 환자와의 의사소통:
- 환자에게 간호 절차를 이해하기 쉬운 언어로 설명했는가?
- 환자의 질문에 성실히 답변하고, 필요한 정보를 제공했는가?
- 환자의 문화적 배경을 존중하며, 적절한 언어와 태도를 사용했는가?

↳ 의료진과의 의사소통:
- 동료 간호사나 의료진에게 환자의 상태를 명확히 보고했는가?
- 정확하고 간결한 문서화를 통해 정보를 효과적으로 전달했는가?

🔖 시간 관리(Time Management)

OSCE는 제한된 시간 내에 간호사가 주어진 과제를 얼마나 효율적으로 완료하는지를 평가합니다. 시간 관리는 실제 임상 현장에서 환자들이 다양한 요구를 할 때, 이를 효과적으로 처리할 수 있는 능력을 평가합니다.

↳ 우선순위 설정:
- 환자의 요구를 사정하고, 중요한 문제를 먼저 해결했는가?
- 응급 상황에서는 신속하고 적절하게 대응했는가?

↳ 효율성:
- 각 단계에서 시간을 적절히 분배하여 모든 과제를 완료했는가?
- 불필요한 절차나 행동을 줄이고, 간결하게 작업을 수행했는가?

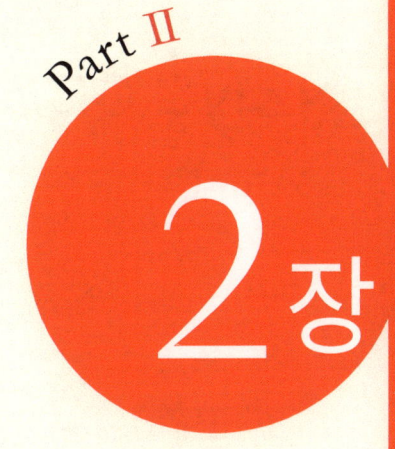

Part II

2장

핵심 간호술기와 10 단계 수행절차,
체크리스트

NZNC OSCE Scenarios

OSCE는 각 스테이션별로 고유한 평가 목표를 가지고 있습니다. 어떤 스테이션에서는 실제 임상 술기를 정확하게 수행하는 것이 중요하고, 또 다른 스테이션에서는 환자와의 효과적인 의사소통 능력을 보여주어야 합니다. 각 스테이션 입장 전 주어지는 2분의 준비 시간을 효율적으로 활용하여 해당 스테이션의 핵심 과제와 평가 포인트를 정확히 파악하는 것이 성공의 열쇠입니다.

OSCE는 해외 간호사 자격 취득을 위한 필수 관문입니다. 이 시험은 단순한 지식 평가를 넘어 실제 임상 현장에서 필요한 종합적인 간호 역량을 평가합니다. 체계적인 이론 학습과 실전 같은 모의 훈련, 그리고 지속적인 피드백을 통한 개선 과정을 거친다면, 충분히 좋은 결과를 얻을 수 있습니다. OSCE에 도전하시는 모든 예비 뉴질랜드 간호사분들의 성공을 진심으로 응원합니다!

이제 부터는 10가지 오스키 스테이션에서 대표적으로 나오는 시나리오를 아래에 영어/한글 버전으로 나열하고, 주요 포인트와 패스하기 쉬운 팁, 마킹 기준을 제시해 드립니다.

Station ❶
Mental Health Assessment

Station ❷
Physiological assessment

Station ❸
Specific physiological assessment

Station ❹
Professional Responsibility

Station ❺
Emergency management

Station ❻
Clinical skills

Station ❼
Medication Administration

Station ❽
Communication and teamwork

Station ❾
Planning nursing care

Station ❿
Managing the deteriorating patient

❶ 정신 건강 사정

Station 1: Mental Health Assessment

✒ 스테이션 목표
- 환자의 심리적 상태를 이해하고 불안증이나 우울증과 같은 정신질환의 징후와 증상을 사정할 수 있다.
- 환자와의 라포(rapport)를 형성하고, 신뢰를 바탕으로 개방적인 대화를 이끌어낸다.
- 환자의 안전을 최우선으로 하여 위급 상황 여부를 평가한다.
- 환자 상태에 따라 적절한 간호 계획과 개입을 제안한다.

✒ 주요 기술

1. 초기 의사소통 및 환경 설정
- 환자에게 본인 소개 후, 면담의 목적과 과정을 설명하여 환자가 안심할 수 있도록 한다.
- 비판단적이고 공감적인 태도로 환자와 대화를 시작하며 라포를 형성.
- 환자와 대화할 때 조용하고 편안한 환경을 제공.

2. 정보 수집(Mental Health Assessment)
- **주관적 데이터 수집:**
  - 환자의 현재 상태(감정, 기분, 걱정거리)를 확인.

- "최근 들어 어떤 기분이 드셨나요?", "가장 걱정되는 것은 무엇인가요?"와 같은 개방형 질문 사용.
↳ **객관적 데이터 수집:**
- 환자의 외모, 행동, 말투, 눈 맞춤 여부 등을 관찰.
- 정신 상태 검사(MSE, Mental State Examination)를 통해 사고 과정, 정서, 집중력 등을 평가.

3. 우울증/불안증 평가
↳ **우울증:** 슬픔, 흥미 상실, 피로감, 집중력 저하, 식욕 변화, 자살 생각 여부 등 확인.
↳ **불안증:** 지나친 걱정, 신체적 증상(심장 두근거림, 발한, 떨림), 공포증 여부 등 확인.
↳ **질문 예시:**
- "평소 즐거웠던 활동에 대한 흥미를 잃으셨나요?"
- "요즘 밤에 잠을 잘 이루시나요?"
- "자신을 해치고 싶은 생각이 드신 적이 있나요?"

4. 안전 사정(Suicide Risk Assessment)
↳ **자살 위험 평가:** "스스로를 해치고 싶다고 느끼신 적이 있나요?" "그럴 때 구체적인 계획이 있었나요?"
↳ 위기 상황 시 병원 프로토콜에 따라 즉각 보고 및 개입 준비.

5. 환자 중심의 의사소통
↳ 환자의 말을 경청하고, 감정을 인정하며 공감하는 태도.
↳ 치료 옵션이나 지원 서비스에 대해 설명하며, 환자의 의견을 반영.
↳ "당신은 혼자가 아니며, 우리가 도움을 드릴 수 있습니다"와 같은 위로와 지지의 말 제공.

> **✱ Tip here!**
>
> 뉴질랜드에서는 환자의 말을 경청하고 공감하며, Reassurance를 제공하는 부분을 정신건강 케어만이 아닌 모든 널싱케어 부분에서 아주 크게 여깁니다. 환자의 말을 끊지 말고 격려, 위로하고 적절한 대안책을 제안하여 환자의 의견을 묻는게 중요합니다.

6. 적절한 문서화
- 환자의 상태, 주요 증상, 의사소통 내용, 사정 결과를 명확히 기록.
- 자살 위험이 있는 경우, 이를 즉시 보고하고 계획된 개입을 문서화.

평가 기준

1. 의사소통 능력
- 라포를 형성하고 비판단적 태도로 환자의 이야기를 경청했는지 평가.
- 개방형 질문과 적극적 경청 기술 사용 여부 확인.

2. 정신 건강 사정 기술
- 우울증/불안증의 주요 증상 및 징후를 정확히 파악했는지 평가.
- 환자의 안전을 최우선으로 하여 자살 위험 여부를 평가했는지 확인.

3. 환자 중심의 간호 접근
- 환자의 감정을 인정하고 공감적 태도를 보였는지 평가.
- 환자가 이해할 수 있도록 적절한 정보 제공 여부 확인.

4. 안전과 적절성
- 위급 상황을 인지하고 병원 프로토콜에 따라 즉각적인 개입을 준비했는지 평가.

5. 시간 관리 및 문서화
- 주어진 시간 안에 사정과 의사소통을 효과적으로 완료했는지 평가.
- 사정 결과와 계획을 정확하게 문서화했는지 확인.

🗒 학습 팁

1. 정신 건강 사정 모델 학습
- Mental State Examination(MSE)와 자살 위험 평가 도구 등을 익혀 반복 연습.

2. 공감 의사소통 기술 연습
- 모의 환자와 시뮬레이션을 통해 공감적이고 비판단적인 의사소통 연습.
- 환자의 말을 반복하며 이해를 확인하는 기술을 사용: "즉, ~라고 말씀하셨던 것 맞나요?"

3. 시나리오 기반 연습
- 우울증, 불안증을 겪는 환자와의 대화 시나리오를 작성하고 실제 상황처럼 연습.
- 자살 위험 평가 시 안전한 환경에서 적절히 대처하는 법을 학습.

4. 문서화 연습
- 사례별로 환자의 상태를 간략하고 명확하게 기록하는 연습을 반복.

5. 스트레스 관리 기술 공유
- 환자에게 심호흡, 점진적 근육 이완 등의 간단한 기술을 소개할 수 있도록 연습.

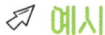 예시

1. Case Description:

A 45-year-old male patient, Mr. David Lee, visits the outpatient clinic. He reports feeling increasingly overwhelmed and fatigued for the past month. During the consultation, he mentions experiencing difficulty sleeping, lack of appetite, and feelings of worthlessness. He states, "I feel like I can't do anything right, and I don't see the point in trying anymore." He avoids eye contact and appears visibly withdrawn.

> 45세 남성 환자 David Lee 씨가 외래 클리닉을 방문했습니다. 그는 지난 한 달 동안 점점 더 스트레스가 쌓이고 피로감을 느꼈다고 호소합니다. 상담 중 그는 잠을 잘 이루지 못하고 식욕이 없으며 무가치함을 느낀다고 말합니다. 그는 "제가 하는 건 전부 잘못인 것 같고, 더 이상 노력할 필요가 없는 것 같아요"라고 말합니다. 그는 눈을 잘 맞추지 않으며 눈에 띄게 위축된 모습입니다.

2. Tasks for the Nurse:

- **2.1** Greet the patient, introduce yourself, and explain the purpose of the assessment.
- **2.2** Build rapport with Mr. Lee and use open-ended questions to explore his emotional and mental state.
- **2.3** Conduct a mental health assessment focusing on mood, thoughts, and risk factors such as self-harm or suicidal ideation.
- **2.4** Offer empathy and support while maintaining a professional and non-judgmental demeanor.
- **2.5** If necessary, develop a care plan, including referrals to mental health specialists.

2.1 환자에게 인사하고, 본인을 소개한 후 사정의 목적을 설명합니다.
2.2 Mr. Lee와 라포(rapport)를 형성하고, 개방형 질문을 사용해 그의 감정 및 정신 상태를 탐색합니다.
2.3 기분, 사고, 자해 또는 자살 생각과 같은 위험 요소를 중심으로 정신 건강 사정을 실시합니다.
2.4 공감과 지지적 간호를 제공하며 전문적이고 비판단적인 태도를 유지합니다.
2.5 필요 시 정신 건강 전문가에게 의뢰를 포함한 간호 계획을 수립합니다.

3. Possible Dialogue Example

Nurse: Hi Mr. Lee, I'm [Your Name], one of the nurses here. It's nice to meet you. How are you feeling today?

Patient: Not so good… I've been feeling really tired and kind of hopeless lately.

Nurse: I'm sorry to hear that, Mr. Lee. That must be really difficult for you. Thank you for being open with me. I'm here to help, and I'd like to ask you a few questions to better understand how you're feeling and what might be causing this. Is that okay with you?

Patient: Yeah, I guess so.

Nurse: Great. Let's start with how long you've been feeling this way. Can you tell me when these feelings started?

Patient: I don't know… maybe a month or so ago? I just started feeling really low, like I can't do anything right.

Nurse: I see. And how has this been affecting your daily life? For example, how are you sleeping? Are you eating regularly?

Patient: Not great. I barely sleep at night. I keep waking up, and when I do manage to fall asleep, I have these bad dreams. I'm not really eating much either… I just don't feel hungry anymore.

Nurse: That sounds exhausting. Sleep and eating are so important for our physical and emotional well-being, so it's understandable that this might be making things feel even harder for you. Have you noticed any changes in your mood during the day? For example, do you feel like things are improving at all, or does it stay the same?

Patient: No, it's just the same all the time. I feel like nothing matters, like there's no point in even trying.

Nurse: That must be really overwhelming to feel that way. Have you ever felt like this before, or is this the first time it's happened?

Patient: I felt a bit like this a few years ago when I lost my job, but it wasn't this bad.

Nurse: Thank you for sharing that with me. It's important that we talk about this, so we can work together to make things feel more manageable for you. Let me ask you one more question, and it might be a little difficult to answer, but it's important. Have you had any thoughts of hurting yourself or feeling like life isn't worth living?

Patient: …Yeah, I've thought about it sometimes, but I don't think I'd actually do anything.

Nurse: I understand, and I really appreciate you being honest with me. It's a brave step to talk about these feelings. I want you to know that you're not alone, and there are people here who care about you and want to help. I'd like to share this with the doctor and our mental health team so we can create a plan to support you. Does that sound okay?

Patient: Yeah… I guess so.

간호사: 안녕하세요, Lee 씨. 저는 여기서 일하는 간호사 [본인 이름]입니다. 만나 뵙게 되어 반갑습니다. 오늘 기분이 어떠신가요?
환자: 별로 좋지 않아요… 요즘 너무 피곤하고 희망이 없는 기분이에요.
간호사: 정말 힘드셨겠어요. 제게 솔직히 말씀해 주셔서 감사합니다. 제가 도와드릴 수 있도록 몇 가지 질문을 드리고 싶어요. 괜찮으신가요?
환자: 네, 괜찮아요.
간호사: 감사합니다. 언제부터 이런 기분이 들기 시작했는지 기억나시나요?
환자: 음… 한 달 정도 된 것 같아요. 그냥 점점 더 기운이 없고, 제가 뭘 해도 다 잘못하는 것 같아요.
간호사: 그렇군요. 이런 기분이 평소 생활에 어떤 영향을 주고 있는지 말씀해 주실 수 있을까요? 예를 들어, 잠은 잘 주무시나요? 식사는 어떻게 하세요?
환자: 별로예요. 밤에 거의 잠을 못 자요. 자꾸 깨고, 간신히 잠들어도 이상한 꿈만 꿔요. 밥도 거의 안 먹고요… 그냥 배고픈 느낌이 안 들어요.

간호사: 정말 많이 지치셨겠어요. 잠과 식사는 몸과 마음 건강에 정말 중요한데, 그게 잘 안 되고 계신다면 더 힘드셨을 것 같아요. 혹시 하루 동안 기분 변화가 있나요? 예를 들어, 어느 때는 나아진다거나 더 나빠진다거나 하는 게 있으신가요?

환자: 아니요, 그냥 항상 똑같아요. 아무 의미도 없고, 뭘 해도 소용없는 것 같아요.

간호사: 그런 감정이 드는 건 정말 힘든 일이겠어요. 혹시 예전에 이런 기분을 느껴본 적이 있으신가요? 아니면 이번이 처음인가요?

환자: 몇 년 전에 직장을 잃었을 때 비슷한 기분이 들었지만, 이번처럼 심하지는 않았어요.

간호사: 말씀해 주셔서 감사합니다. 이런 이야기를 나누는 건 정말 중요해요. 이제 한 가지 질문을 더 드리고 싶은데, 조금 어려운 질문일 수 있지만 중요한 내용이에요. 혹시 스스로를 해치고 싶다거나, 삶이 가치 없다고 느끼신 적이 있으신가요?

환자: ...네, 가끔 그런 생각을 해요. 근데 제가 실제로 뭘 하지는 않을 것 같아요.

간호사: 이해합니다. 이렇게 솔직히 말씀해 주셔서 정말 감사드려요. 이런 감정을 이야기하는 건 용기가 필요한 일이에요. Lee 씨는 혼자가 아니시고, 여기에는 Lee 씨를 걱정하고 도와드리고 싶어 하는 사람들이 있어요. 이 내용을 담당 의사와 정신건강팀과 공유해서 Lee 씨를 지원할 계획을 세우고 싶습니다. 괜찮으실까요?

환자: 네... 그러세요.

Key Elements in Dialogue:

1. Empathy and validation of the patient's feelings.
2. Open-ended questions to explore mood, thoughts, and behavior.
3. Assessing risk factors like self-harm or suicidal ideation with sensitivity.
4. Offering support and explaining the next steps clearly to reassure the patient.

📌 마킹 기준 체크리스트 Marking Criteria

Category	Step	Met	Not Met
1. Preparation			
Ensure the environment is safe and private	Confirm the setting is conducive to open communication and respect patient confidentiality		
Gather necessary information and materials	Review patient history or referral notes before starting the assessment		
Establish rapport	Introduce yourself, confirm the patient's identity and explain the purpose of the assessment		
2. Mental Health Assessment			
Assess the patient's appearance and behaviour	Observe and document hygiene, posture, eye contact, and mannerisms		
Evaluate mood and affect	Ask about the patient's current feelings and observe their emotional state		
Screen for suicidal or self harming thoughts	Directly ask about thoughts of self-harm or suicide in a sensitive manner		
Assess thought process and content	Evaluate for signs of delusions, hallucinations, or disorganised thinking		
Screen for risk factors	Identify risks related to harm to self, and others, or inability to care for oneself		
Assess orientation and cognition	Check for orientation to person, place and time as well as memory and concentration		
3. Communication skills			

Use active listening skills	Demonstrate alternativeness through verbal and non-verbal cues(e.g. nodding, maintaining eye contact)		
Ask open-ended and non-judgemental questions	Encourage the patient to share freely without feeling pressured		
Respond empathetically	Validate the patient's feelings and concerns in a supportive manner		
Paraphrases and summarise	Reflect back key points to ensure understanding and clarity		
Maintain professionalism	Demonstrate respect, patience, and cultural sensitivity throughout		
4. Documentation and Handover			
Summarise findings clearly	Provide a concise and accurate summary of the assessment outcomes		
Develop an action plan	Identify immediate actions, follow-up care, or referrals as needed		
Complete documentation accurately	Record key findings in the appropriate format		
Communicate findings effectively	Share relevant information with team members or supervisors in a professional manner		
5. Professionalism			
Adhere to ethical and legal standards	Maintain confidentiality and ensure informed consent is obtained where necessary		
Demonstrate cultural competence	Acknowledge and respect cultural differences in communication and care		
Manage time effectively	Complete the assessment and communication within the allocated time frame		

② 신체사정(활력징후 측정)

Station two: Physiological assessment

✒ 스테이션 목표
- 환자의 기본 활력징후(혈압, 맥박, 호흡수, 체온, 산소포화도)를 정확히 측정하고, 결과를 해석하여 환자의 상태를 평가할 수 있다.
- 측정 과정에서 환자와 효과적으로 소통하며, 절차를 안전하고 위생적으로 수행한다.

✒ 주요기술

1. 손 위생 및 PPE 착용:
- 모든 측정 전에 손 위생을 철저히 하고 필요 시 개인 보호 장비(PPE)를 착용합니다.

2. 혈압 측정:
- 적절한 크기의 커프 선택.
- 예상 수축기 혈압을 측정한 후 정확한 혈압 측정.
- 무음 간격(Auscultatory Gap) 인지.

3. 맥박 측정:
- 요골동맥이나 경동맥에서 맥박을 정확히 측정.
- 속도, 리듬, 강도를 평가.

4. 호흡수 측정:
- 환자가 인지하지 못하도록 자연스럽게 호흡수를 측정.
- 분당 호흡수와 규칙성, 깊이를 평가.

5. 체온 측정:
- 체온계를 사용하는 방법에 따라(구강, 액와, 고막, 직장) 정확히 측정.

6. 산소포화도 측정:
- 펄스옥시미터를 적절히 사용하여 산소포화도 확인.
- 결과 해석 및 필요 시 추가 평가.

7. 결과 기록:
- 정확한 활력징후 수치를 환자 기록지에 작성.
- 정상 범위를 벗어난 경우 즉각 보고.

평가기준

1. 손 위생 및 PPE 착용 여부를 확인.
2. 각 활력징후를 정확하고 안전하게 측정하는지 관찰.
3. 장비 사용 방법이 적절한지 평가(예: 혈압 커프 위치와 크기, 체온계 사용 방법 등).
4. 활력징후 결과를 정확히 기록하고, 임상적으로 해석하는지 평가.
5. 환자와의 의사소통 및 설명 능력을 평가.
6. 과정을 마친 후 손 위생을 수행했는지 확인.

학습팁

1. **장비 사용법 숙지**: 혈압계, 체온계, 펄스옥시미터 등 주요 장비의 작동법을 숙달하세요.
2. **정상 범위 암기**: 각 활력징후의 정상 범위를 기억하고, 비정상적인 결과가 무엇을 의미하는지 공부하세요.

3. **체계적인 접근법 연습**: 항상 동일한 순서로 활력징후를 측정하여 실수 없이 정확히 수행할 수 있도록 합니다(예: 체온 → 맥박 → 호흡수 → 혈압 → 산소포화도).
4. **환자와의 소통 연습**: 활력징후를 측정하는 동안 환자에게 명확히 설명하고, 불편을 최소화하세요.
5. **시간 관리**: 제한된 시간 안에 모든 측정을 완료할 수 있도록 연습하세요.
6. **피드백 받기**: 동료나 강사로부터 피드백을 받아 개선점을 파악하세요.

예시

1. Preparation

Hand sanitises before the procedure or touching the patient and ensure that all necessary equipment is available and functioning correctly. Equipment needed includes:

> 활력징후 측정전이나 환자를 터치 하기 전에 손을 소독하고 필요한 장비가 모두 작동 중인지 확인하세요. 필요한 장비는 다음과 같습니다:

Tip here!

> 손 소독은 의료관련감염을 예방하고 환자 안전을 위한 가장 기본적이고 효과적인 방법입니다. OSCE에서 손소독 수행은 간호사의 기본적인 임상 능력과 전문성을 평가하는 중요한 항목입니다.

1.1 Thermometer 체온계
1.2 Blood pressure cuff 혈압측정기
1.3 Stethoscope 청진기
1.4 Watch or timer 시계 혹은 타이머
1.5 Pen and documentation chart 펜과 문서화 차트

2. Introduction yourself and Consent: 본인소개및 동의

2.1 Knock on the door before entering.

> 방에 들어가기전 노크를 합니다.

2.2 Greet the patient: "Hello, my name is [Your Name], and I am a registered nurse, looking after you today. Today, I'd like to take your vital signs, which include your blood pressure, temperature, heart rate, and respiratory rate. This will only take a few minutes. Is that okay with you?"

> 환자에게 인사: "안녕하세요, 제 이름은 [본인 이름]이고, 저는 오늘 환자분을 간호할 간호사입니다. 오늘은 혈압, 체온, 심박수, 호흡수를 포함한 활력 징후를 측정하려고 합니다. 몇 분 정도 소요됩니다. 괜찮으신가요?"

✳ Tip here!

> 간호사로서 의료행위를 하기전 환자의 동의를 받는것은 아주 큰 첫번째 스텝입니다.(특히 뉴질랜드 널싱에서 아주 중시 하는 부분) 이는 환자의 자기 결정권을 존중하고 자신이 받을 의료행위에 대해 충분히 고려하고 결정할 권리가 있음을 인정해 주는것입니다. 이는 또한 환자~의료인 사이의 의사소통을 촉진하고 상호신뢰를 높입니다. 따라서 활력증후 측정 전 환자의 동의를 구하는 것은 환자의 권리를 존중하고, 의료의 질을 높이며, 법적, 윤리적 의무를 이행하는 중요한 과정입니다.

2.3 Verify patient identity: "Can you please confirm your full name and date of birth?"

> 환자 신원 확인: "성함과 생년월일을 확인해 주시겠어요?"

2.4 Explain the process briefly: "I will take measurements one by one, starting with your temperature."

과정 간단히 설명: "체온 측정부터 시작하여 하나씩 측정하겠습니다."

2.5 Ensure the patient is comfortable and appropriately positioned.

환자가 편안하고 적절히 자세를 잡도록 도와주세요.

3. Step-by-Step Procedure:
3.1 Measure Temperature: 체온측정
- Use the appropriate thermometer in the station(oral, tympanic, or temporal).

오스키 스테이션에서 주어진 적절한 체온계(구강, 고막, 이마)를 사용하세요.

- If using an ear thermometer: 고막 체온계 사용시
  - Ask if it is ok to touch their head and ears.

  (Māori culture relation)

환자에게 그들의 머리와 귀를 만져도 되는지 물어보세요.

 Tip here!

뉴질랜드 널싱시 중요시 여겨야 하는것중 하나가 개인의 존엄성을 인정하고 동의를 구하는 것입니다. 특히 마오리 문화의 맥락에서 환자의 귀 체온을 측정할 때 머리를 만져도 되는지 물어보는 것은 아주 결정적인 질문입니다. 마오리 문화에서 머리는 매우 신성하고 중요한 부위로 여겨집니다. 따라서 허락 없이 타인의 머리를 만지는 것은 무례할 수 있습니다. 그러하여 이러한 문화적 민감성을 보여주는 것은 의료진의 문화적 역량을 반영하며, 더 나은 환자 케어로 이어질 수 있습니다.

- Make sure to pull the ear back and up prior to insertion of the thermometer

체온계 삽입전, 귀를 위로 그리고 뒤로 잡아 당기는 점을 명심하세요.

- Wait for the thermometer to beep or indicate it has completed the reading.

체온계가 신호음이 나거나 측정 완료를 표시할 때까지 기다립니다.

- Record the reading accurately.

정확히 기록하세요.

3.2 Measure Pulse: 맥박측정

↬ Ask the patient to relax their arm and position it palm-up.

환자가 팔을 편안히 놓고 손바닥을 위로 향하게 하세요.

↬ Locate the **radial pulse**(on the thumb side of the wrist).

요골 동맥(손목의 엄지손가락 쪽)을 찾으세요.

↬ Use the pads of your index and middle fingers to apply gentle pressure.

검지와 중지로 부드럽게 압력을 가하세요.

↳ **Count the beats for 30 seconds and multiply by 2** to get the beats per minute(BPM). If the pulse is irregular, count for a full 60 seconds.

30초 동안 박동을 세고 2를 곱하여 분당 박동수(BPM)를 계산하세요. 맥박이 불규칙한 경우 60초 동안 세도록 하세요.

↳ Note the rhythm(regular/irregular) and pulse strength.

리듬(규칙적/불규칙적)과 강도를 기록하세요.

3.3 Measure Respiratory Rate: 호흡수 측정
↳ While appearing to take the pulse, discreetly observe the patient's chest rise and fall.

맥박을 측정하는 척하면서 환자의 흉부 상승과 하강을 관찰하세요.

↳ Count the number of breaths(one inhalation and exhalation equals one breath) **for 1 mins.**

숨을 들이쉬고 내쉬는 것을 한 번으로 계산하여 1분동안 호흡수를 계산하세요.

↳ Record whether the breathing is regular or irregular and note any abnormalities(e.g., laboured breathing).

호흡이 규칙적인지 불규칙적인지 기록하고 비정상적인 점(예: 힘든 호흡)이 있는지 확인하세요.

3.4 Measure Blood Pressure: 혈압측정

➣ Ensure the patient is seated comfortably with their arm supported at heart level and feet flat on the floor.

> 환자가 편안히 앉아 있고 팔이 심장 높이에서 지지되며 발이 바닥에 평평하게 놓여 있는지 확인하세요.

➣ **Choose the right size cuff** for the patient's arm.

> 환자의 팔에 맞는 사이즈의 커프를 고르세요.

➣ Using a manual cuff:
  - Place the stethoscope's diaphragm over the brachial artery.

> 청진기의 다이어프램을 상완 동맥 위에 놓으세요.

  - Inflate the cuff to 20-30 mmHg above the patient's estimated systolic pressure(if known) or 180 mmHg.

> 커프를 환자의 예상 수축기압(알고 있는 경우)보다 20-30 mmHg 높이거나 180 mmHg까지 팽창시키세요.

(✱) Tip here!

> 혈압을 측정할 때 예상 수축기압을 측정하는 것이 약간의 시간이 추가로 소비된다는 단점이 있기는 하지만 OSCE는 candidates의 정확한 기술과 절차 준수를 평가하는 시험입니다. 예상 수축기 혈압을 먼저 측정하는 방법은 무음 간격(Auscultatory Gap) 으로 인한 오류를 방지하므로, 정확한 혈압 수치를 기록할 수 있고 간호사가 **표준화된 절차(Standardized Procedure)**를 준수하고 있는지 평가 할수 있는 잣대이기도 합니다.

- Slowly release the pressure(2-3 mmHg per second) and listen for Korotkoff sounds.
  · The first sound indicates the systolic pressure.
  · The point where the sound disappears indicates the diastolic pressure.

> 압력을 천천히 해제하세요(초당 2-3 mmHg) 그리고 Korotkoff 소리를 들으세요.
> · 첫 번째 소리가 수축기압을 나타냅니다.
> · 소리가 사라지는 지점이 이완기압을 나타냅니다.

- Record the reading as systolic/diastolic(e.g., 120/80 mmHg).

> 수치를 수축기/이완기 형태로 기록하세요(예: 120/80 mmHg).

3.5 Document Findings: 결과 문서화

↪ Accurately record all vital signs in the patient's chart or documentation tool:

> 환자의 차트에 모든 활력징후를 정확히 기록하세요.

- Temperature(e.g., 36.8°C oral)
- Pulse(e.g., 72 BPM, regular)
- Respiratory rate(e.g., 16 breaths per minute, regular)
- Blood pressure(e.g., 120/80 mmHg, seated)

↪ Make sure to document - Date, time and signature and role

> 날짜, 시간, 이름과 직책을 꼭 기록하세요.

4. Closing the Procedure: 절차 마무리

➢ Thank the patient: "Thank you for your cooperation. Do you have any questions or concerns?"

> 환자에게 감사 인사: "협조해 주셔서 감사합니다. 질문이나 걱정되는 점이 있으신가요?"

➢ Ensure the patient is comfortable.

> 환자가 편안한 상태인지 확인하세요.

➢ Sanitize your hands

> 손을 소독하세요

➢ Clean and store equipment properly.

> 장비를 깨끗이 정리하고 보관하세요.

Common Errors to Avoid

1. Failing to sanitize hands before and after the procedure.
   * 절차 전후에 손을 소독하지 않는 것.
2. Incorrect equipment placement (e.g., stethoscope, cuff, thermometer).
   * 잘못된 방법으로 청진기나 커프, 체온계를 사용하는것.

3. Miscounting or estimating pulse and respiratory rates.
   * 맥박및 호흡수를 잘못 세거나 추정해서 노트에 남기는것
4. Failing to communicate findings or abnormalities promptly.
   * 결과나 이상점을 즉시 전달하지 않는것
5. Not recognizing the specific element to focus on and respond appropriately to the patient based on the scenario.
   * 시나리오를 바탕으로 집중해야 할 특정 요소를 인식하지 못한채 환자에게 적절한 대답을 하지 못하는것.

마킹 기준 체크리스트 Marking Criteria

Category	Step	Met	Not Met
1. Preparation			
Introduce yourself and your role	"Hello, my name is(Name) and I am your nurse today"		
Wash hands or use hand sanitiser	Use proper hand hygiene before staring the procedure		
Confirm patient identity	Ask for the patient's full name and DOB, and check the wristband if applicable		
Explain the procedure	Clearly explain what will happen and gain verbal consent		
Gather and prepare equipment	Ensure all equipment is present and functional		
2. Measuring Temperature			
Select appropriate thermometer	Use proper thermometer based on the station		

Place thermometer accurately	Ensure proper technique is used. ex. Pull up and back for ear thermometer		
Wait appropriate time	Wait for the device to signal completion or reads mercury thermometer at correct time		
Record temperature accurately	Documents the value accurately		
3. Measuring Pulse			
Locate radial pulse	Place index and middle fingers on the wrist		
Count pulse for appropriate time	Count for 30 sec and multiplies by 2		
Record pulse accurately	Document rate and rhythm		
4. Measuring respiratory rate			
Observe chest movement discreetly	Ensure the patient is unaware to prevent altered breathing patterns		
Count respirations	Count breaths for 1 minute		
Assess respiratory effort if necessary	Note depth(shallow/deep) and effort(laboured/unlaboured)		
Record respiratory rate accurately	Document rate, depth, and effort		
5. Measuring blood pressure			
Select appropriate cuff size	Ensure the cuff size is suitable for the patient's arm		
Positions patient correctly	Ensure the patient is seated or lying, with arm at heart level and relaxed		
Locate brachial artery	Palpate brachial artery and position cuff correctly above the artery		
Inflate cuff to appropriate pressure	Inflate 20-30mmhg above the estimated systolic BP		

Deflate cuff slowly and steadily	Listen for Korotkoff sounds while deflating at 2-3 mmHg per second		
Record systolic and diastolic readings	Document accurately		
Remove cuff and ensure patient comfort	Remove the cuff gently and reassure the patient		
6. Measuring oxygen saturation(Spo2)			
Attach pulse oximeter correctly	Place the probe on a finger free of nail polish or obstruction		
Waits for stable reading	Ensure the device gives a stable and accurate reading.(e.g. ask the patient to minimise the movement)		
Record oxygen saturation accurately	Document value and any relevant observation.(e.g : spo2 98% on room air)		
7. Post-procedure			
Ensure patient comfort	Ask the patient if they are comfortable and address any concerns		
Clean and store equipment	Disinfect reusable equipment and store it properly		
Wash hands or use hand sanitiser	Perform hand hygiene after completing the procedure		
Document all findings accurately	Complete documentation clearly, accurately and promptly		
8. Professionalism			
Demonstrate respectful communication	Maintain professionalism and use appropriate language throughout.		
Manage time effectively	Complete the task efficiently within the allowed time		

❸ 세부 생리학적 사정

Station Three: Specific physiological assessment
Assessing a patient with a Cast for Compartment Syndrome

⚘ 스테이션 목표

- 석고붕대를 가진 환자의 구획증후군(compartment syndrome) 발생 가능성을 조기에 사정하는 능력을 평가합니다.
- 환자의 신경혈관 상태(neurovascular status)를 체계적으로 평가하여, 잠재적인 이상징후를 식별하고 적시에 적절한 간호 및 보고를 시행합니다.
- 환자와의 명확하고 효과적인 의사소통을 통해 환자의 안위를 보장하며, 치료적 관계를 유지합니다.
- 팀워크와 상황 대응 능력을 통해 환자 중심의 간호를 제공하고, 응급 상황을 예방할수 있어야 합니다.

⚘ 주요 기술

1. 신경혈관 사정 기술:

- **6P 평가:** 구획 증후군의 주요 징후인 통증(Pain), 창백(Pallor), 감각 이상(Paraesthesia), 마비(Paralysis), 맥박 소실(Pulselessness), 냉기(Poikilothermia)을 체계적으로 사정.
- 석고붕대 주변의 피부 상태 관찰: 부종, 붉은 반점, 냉기 또는 피부 긴장 여부 확인.

- 환자에게 통증 수준(0-10)을 묻고, 지속적이고 완화되지 않는 통증 여부 확인.
- 손발의 운동성과 감각을 확인하며, 차가운 느낌이나 무감각(저린 느낌)이 있는지 질문.
- 석고붕대 아래의 압박감 또는 단단한 느낌이 있는지 조심스럽게 검사.

2. 효과적인 의사소통 기술:
- 환자에게 사정의 목적과 과정에 대해 사전에 설명하여 불안감을 완화.

> 예: "Brown 씨, 오늘 제가 당신의 다리에 석고붕대가 잘 맞고 있는지, 그리고 구획 증후군의 증상이 없는지 확인하려고 합니다. 조금 불편할 수 있지만 짧게 끝낼 테니 걱정하지 마세요."

- 사정 중 발견된 징후에 대해 환자와 보호자에게 명확히 설명하고, 추가 조치 계획을 논의.

> 예: "현재 약간의 부종과 통증이 보이는데, 이것은 문제가 될 수 있습니다. 즉시 의사와 상의하여 필요한 조치를 취하겠습니다."

- 환자에게 협조를 요청하며, 통증이나 불편함이 있으면 즉시 알리도록 안내.

3. 긴급 대처 및 보고 기술:
- 구획 증후군이 의심될 경우, 즉각적으로 의료 팀(의사)에게 보고.
- 필요한 경우 석고붕대를 제거하거나 느슨하게 할 수 있도록 의사의 지시에 따름.
- 발견 사항과 시행 조치를 정확히 문서화.
- 환자의 상태가 악화되지 않도록 지속적으로 관찰하며, 후속 조치를 실행.

4. 윤리적 배려 및 안전 기술:
- 환자의 사생활과 존엄성을 보호하며, 사정 중 적절한 프라이버시 제공.
- 석고붕대와 주변 부위를 만질 때 감염 예방을 위해 손 위생을 철저히 시행.

평가기준

1. 사정 정확성: 6P를 포함한 신경혈관 사정을 체계적이고 정확하게 수행했는가?

2. 의사소통: 환자와 보호자에게 명확하고 친절한 설명을 제공하며, 필요한 협조를 요청했는가?

3. 응급 대처: 구획 증후군의 징후가 의심되는 경우, 즉시 보고 및 적절한 조치를 시행했는가?

4. 문서화: 사정 결과와 후속 조치를 적시에 기록했는가?

5. 환자 안전: 사정 중 환자의 안전과 안위를 고려하며, 감염 예방 조치를 시행했는가?

학습 팁

1. 구획 증후군에 대한 이해
- 구획 증후군의 원인, 병리 생리학, 그리고 주요 징후 및 증상을 심도 있게 학습하기.
- 석고붕대 적용 환자에서 발생할 수 있는 신경혈관 손상과 그 결과를 이해하기.

2. 신경혈관 사정 연습
- 시뮬레이션 환경에서 반복적으로 6P 평가를 연습하기.
- 부위별 사정 방법(팔/다리)을 구분하여 정확히 시행하는 기술을 익히기.
- 시간 내에 체계적으로 사정을 완료하는 능력을 기르기.

3. 효과적인 의사소통 개발
- 환자에게 친근하고 신뢰감을 주는 대화를 연습하기.
- 어려운 상황(통증 호소, 불안감)이 있는 환자에게 대처하는 방법을 학습하기.

4. 응급 상황 대응 능력 강화
- 구획 증후군이 의심될 때 필요한 초기 조치와 보고 방법을 반복적으로 연습하기.
- 의료 팀과의 협업 시뮬레이션을 통해 보고 및 대처 과정을 익히기.

5. 문서화 능력 향상
- 사정 결과, 조치 계획, 그리고 환자의 반응을 간결하고 명확하게 기록하는 방법을 학습하기.
- 문서화 시 놓치기 쉬운 세부 정보를 확인하는 체크리스트를 만들어 활용하기.

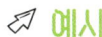 예시

1. Case description:

Mr. Brown is a patient who has had a cast applied to his right leg for 24 hours and is complaining of persistent pain and swelling in the leg. The patient reports that the pain is not subsiding and mentions a decreased sensation in the toes.

> Brown 씨는 오른쪽 다리에 석고붕대를 적용받은 지 24시간이 된 환자로, 지속적인 통증과 다리의 부종을 호소합니다. 환자는 통증이 완화되지 않으며, 발가락의 감각이 저하된 느낌이 든다고 말합니다.

2. Tasks for the Nurse:

2.1 Perform a focused assessment for compartment syndrome:

- Assess for the "6P's" of compartment syndrome: Pain (disproportionate to the injury), Pallor, Pulselessness, Paraesthesia(numbness/tingling) ,Paralysis and Poikilothermia(tightness).
- Evaluate the cast for tightness and check the skin condition around the cast.

> - 구획 증후군의 "6가지 P"를 평가합니다: 통증(부상에 비해 과도한 통증), 창백, 맥박 소실, 감각 이상(무감각/저림), 마비, 냉기.
> - 석고붕대의 조임 상태를 확인하고 석고붕대 주변 피부 상태를 점검합니다.

2.2 Document and escalate:

- Record the patient's symptoms and findings accurately.

- Notify the attending doctor or healthcare provider immediately with a clear and concise report using a structured communication tool like ISBAR (Identification Situation, Background, Assessment, Recommendation).

- 환자의 증상과 평가 내용을 정확히 기록합니다.
- 신원확인, 상황, 배경, 평가, 권장(ISBAR)과 같은 구조화된 보고 도구를 사용하여 주치의나 의료진에게 즉시 알립니다.

2.3 Provide appropriate care:
- Reassure the patient and provide comfort measures (e.g., elevating the limb to reduce swelling, if safe to do so).
- Prepare the patient for further interventions, such as loosening the cast or surgical evaluation, as per the doctor's instructions.

- 환자를 안심시키고 편안함을 제공하는 조치를 합니다(예: 부종을 줄이기 위해 사지를 높이는 것, 안전한 경우에 한함).
- 의사의 지시에 따라 석고붕대를 느슨하게 하거나 외과적 평가를 위한 준비를 합니다.

2.4 Monitor continuously:
- Keep monitoring the patient for worsening symptoms or signs of neurovascular compromise.

신경혈관 상태의 악화를 나타내는 증상이나 징후를 지속적으로 관찰합니다.

1) 환자에게 현재 상황을 설명하고 신경혈관 사정을 시작.
   - "Brown 씨, 다리에 불편함이 있다는 말씀 들었습니다. 다리의 혈액순환과 신경 상태를 점검하려고 합니다."
2) 다리의 부종, 창백, 냉기를 확인하고, 발가락의 움직임과 감각을 검사.
   - 발가락의 색깔이 창백하고, 환자가 저린 느낌을 지속적으로 호소.
3) 즉시 담당 의사에게 상황 보고.
   - "Brown 씨의 다리에 부종과 창백이 있으며, 발가락의 감각이 저하되고 있습니다. 구획 증후군이 의심됩니다. 석고붕대의 압박을 완화하거나 추가 검사가 필요합니다."
4) 환자와 보호자에게 현재 상황을 설명하고, 환자의 안위를 보장하며 후속 조치를 이행.

문서화:
↝ "오른쪽 다리 석고붕대 적용 부위에서 지속적인 통증, 부종, 창백, 감각 저하가 관찰됨. 구획 증후군 의심되어 담당 의사에게 보고하였으며, 환자 상태를 지속적으로 모니터링 중임."

📌 마킹 기준 체크리스트 Marking Criteria

Category	Step	Met	Not Met
1. Initial Preparation			
Introduce yourself and your role	"Hello, my name is(Name) and I am your nurse today"		
Wash hands or use hand sanitiser	Use proper hand hygiene before staring the procedure, follow infection prevention protocols		
Confirm patient identity	Ask for the patient's full name and DOB, and check the wristband if applicable		
Explain the procedure of the assessment to the patient	Clearly explain what will happen and gain verbal consent, ensure patient autonomy and informed participation		
2. Observation and inspection			
Observe the cast for signs of tightness or damage	Check for cracks, swelling around the edges or improper fit		
Inspect the affected limb for visible swelling, discolouration, or signs of reduced circulation	Observe for any abnormal changes in the limb		
Note any drainage or odour around the cast site	Assess for potential signs of infection		
3. Pain assessment			
Ask the patient about the location, intensity and nature of the pain	Use a pain scale(e,g,0-10) and assess for disproportionate pain. Pain assessment framework e.g. COLDSPA Character, onset, location, duration, severity, pattern, Associated factors		

Note whether the pain worsens with passive stretch of the limb	Key symptom of compartment syndrome		
4. Neurovascular assessment			
Check for a pulse distal to the cast(e.g., dorsalis pedis, radial pulse)	Assess circulation to the affected area		
Evaluate capillary refill time(should be <2 secs)	Identify any delays in perfusion		
Assess limb temperature by comparing it to the unaffected side	Cold skin may indicate compromised circulation		
Check for sensation in the affected limb	Ask the patient about numbness or tingling sensation		
Assess motor function by asking the patient to move their fingers or toes	Identify any motor deficits		
5. Key signs of Compartment Syndrome			
Identify the 6P's: pain, pallor, pulselessness, paraesthesia, paralysis, Poikilothermia	Demonstrate a thorough understanding of compartment syndrome		
Assess for tense or tight skin around the affected area	Indicate increased pressure within the compartment		

6. Communication and Documentation			
Clearly communicate findings to the patient	Explain results in understandable terms to the patient		
Document all findings accurately and thoroughly	Include all observations, neurovascular checks and pain assessments		
Immediately report any signs of compartment syndrome to the doctor	Ensure prompt escalation to prevent complications		
7. Patient Education			
Ensure the patient about the signs and symptoms of compartment syndrome	Advise the patient to report severe pain, numbness or swelling immediately		
Provide instructions on limb elevation to reduce swelling	Promote circulation and decrease pressure in the limb		
Advise the patient to avoid inserting objects into the cast	Prevent damage to the skin or cast		
8. Professionalism			
Maintain a calm, compassionate, and professional demeanour	Demonstrate confidence and patient-centred care		
Adhere to hospital protocols and safety guidelines	Follow established clinical practices		

④ 전문적인 답변

Station Four: Professional Responsibility
Respecting Māori Patient Decisions and Family-centred Care

🡕 스테이션 목표

🡕 Demonstrate respect for the cultural values, beliefs, and decisions of Māori patients and their whānau (family).

> 마오리 환자와 그들의 가족(whānau)의 문화적 가치, 신념, 결정을 존중하는 것을 보여줍니다.

🡕 Provide care that aligns with the principles of Te Tiriti o Waitangi(The Treaty of Waitangi), including partnership, protection, and participation.

> Te Tiriti o Waitangi(와이탕이 조약)의 원칙(파트너십, 보호, 참여)에 부합하는 간호를 제공합니다.

🡕 Effectively engage and communicate with the patient and their whanau to support shared decision-making.

> 환자와 가족과 효과적으로 소통하여 공동 의사결정을 지원합니다.

↳ Ensure culturally safe practice by incorporating Māori health perspectives and family-centered care principles.

> 마오리 건강 관점과 가족 중심의 간호 원칙을 통합하여 문화적으로 안전한 간호를 보장합니다.

✈ 주요기술

1. Cultural Competency: 문화적 역량

↳ Show awareness and respect for Māori values, including mana(dignity), wairua(spirituality), and whānau involvement in decision-making.

> 마오리의 가치(예: mana(존엄성), wairua(영성), whānau(가족 참여))에 대한 이해와 존중을 보여줍니다.

2. Effective Communication: 효과적인 의사소통

↳ Use culturally appropriate greetings and language, such as "Kia ora" or "Tēnā koe."

> "Kia ora"(안녕하세요), "Tēnā koe"(당신에게 평안을)와 같은 문화적으로 적절한 인사를 사용합니다.

↳ Listen actively to the patient and their whānau to understand their concerns, wishes, and values.

> 환자와 그 가족의 걱정, 소망, 가치를 이해하기 위해 적극적으로 경청합니다.

↳ Avoid judgmental or dismissive language, ensuring empathy and respect throughout the interaction.

공감과 존중을 바탕으로 판단적이거나 무례한 표현을 피합니다.

3. Family-centred Care: 가족중심의 간호

↳ Involve the patient's whānau in care planning and decision-making, recognizing the importance of collective well-being.

환자의 가족을 간호 계획과 의사결정 과정에 포함하며, 집단적인 웰빙의 중요성을 인식합니다.

↳ Provide a safe and welcoming environment for the whānau, allowing their input and support during care delivery.

가족의 의견과 지원을 환영하는 안전하고 환영받는 환경을 제공합니다.

4. Collaboration and Advocacy: 협력 및 옹호

↳ Partner with the patient and their whānau to co-create a care plan that respects their values and preferences.

환자와 가족과 협력하여 그들의 가치와 선호를 존중하는 간호 계획을 공동으로 수립합니다.

↳ Advocate for the patient's decisions and rights within the healthcare team, ensuring cultural safety.

환자의 결정과 권리를 옹호하며 의료 팀 내에서 문화적 안전을 보장합니다.

5. Adherence to Te Tiriti o Waitangi: 와이탕이 조약 원칙 준수

➢ Apply the principles of partnership, protection, and participation in all aspects of care.

> 간호의 모든 측면에서 파트너십, 보호, 참여의 원칙을 적용합니다.

➢ Ensure equitable access to healthcare and honor the patient's cultural identity.

> 의료 서비스의 형평성을 보장하며 환자의 문화적 정체성을 존중합니다.

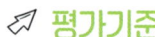 평가기준

1. Cultural Awareness: 문화적 인식

➢ Did the candidate demonstrate understanding and respect for Māori cultural values and practices?

> Candidate가 마오리의 문화적 가치와 관행에 대한 이해와 존중을 보여주었습니까?

➢ Were culturally appropriate greetings and communication used?

> 문화적으로 적절한 인사 및 의사소통이 사용되었습니까?

2. Patient and Whānau Engagement: 환자 및 가족 참여

➢ Was the patient and their whānau actively involved in decision-making?

> 환자와 가족이 의사결정에 적극적으로 참여하도록 했습니까?

↳ Did the candidate create a supportive and non-judgmental environment?

> Candidate가 지지적이고 판단 없는 환경을 만들었습니까?

3. Culturally Safe Care: 문화적으로 안전한 간호

↳ Were the patient's decisions, including the use of traditional Māori practices, respected?

> 전통적인 마오리 관행 사용을 포함하여 환자의 결정이 존중되었습니까?

↳ Did the candidate avoid imposing their own beliefs or preferences on the patient?

> Candidate가 자신의 신념이나 선호를 환자에게 강요하지 않았습니까?

4. Communication: 의사소통

↳ Was the candidate empathetic, clear, and respectful in their communication with the patient and whānau?

> Candidate가 환자와 가족에게 공감적이고 명확하며 존중하는 방식으로 의사소통했습니까?

↳ Did they demonstrate active listening and respond appropriately to concerns?

> 적극적으로 경청하고 적절히 반응했습니까?

5. Adherence to Te Tiriti o Waitangi: 와이탕기 조약 준수

↳ Were the principles of partnership, protection, and participation evident in the candidate's actions?

> Candidate의 행동에서 파트너십, 보호, 참여의 원칙이 나타났습니까?

↳ Did the candidate ensure equitable and culturally safe care?

> Candidate가 형평성 있고 문화적으로 안전한 간호를 보장했습니까?

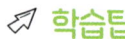 학습팁

1. Learn Key Māori Concepts: 주요 마오리 개념 학습

↳ Understand fundamental Māori values such as mana, wairua, whānau, and tikanga(customs).

> mana(존엄성), wairua(영성), whānau(가족), tikanga(관습) 등 마오리의 기본 가치를 이해합니다.

↳ Familiarize yourself with common Māori terms used in healthcare settings.

> 의료 환경에서 사용되는 일반적인 마오리 용어에 익숙해집니다.

2. Practice Culturally Safe Communication: 문화적으로 안전한 의사소통 연습

↳ Role-play interactions with Māori patients and whānau to practice culturally respectful language and active listening.

> 마오리 환자 및 가족과의 상호작용을 롤플레이하며 문화적으로 존중하는 언어와 경청 기술을 연습합니다.

↳ Use empathetic and non-judgmental phrases, focusing on building trust and rapport.

> 신뢰와 친밀감을 형성하는 공감적이고 판단 없는 표현을 사용합니다.

3. Understand Te Tiriti o Waitangi Principles: 와이탕기 원칙 이해

↳ Study the principles of partnership, protection, and participation and how they apply to healthcare.

> 파트너십, 보호, 참여 원칙을 공부하고 이를 의료 환경에 적용하는 방법을 익힙니다.

↳ Be prepared to explain how your actions align with these principles.

> 본인의 행동이 이러한 원칙에 어떻게 부합하는지 설명할 준비를 합니다.

4. Family-centred Care Practice: 가족중심의 간호 연습

↳ Practice scenarios where whānau are involved in care planning and decision-making.

> 가족이 간호 계획과 의사결정 과정에 포함되는 시나리오를 연습합니다.

↳ Demonstrate flexibility in accommodating family needs and preferences.

가족의 필요와 선호를 수용하는 유연성을 보여줍니다.

5. Cultural Safety Training: 문화적 안전 교육

➢ Attend workshops or online courses on cultural competency and Māori health to deepen your understanding.

문화적 역량과 마오리 건강에 대한 이해를 심화시키기 위해 워크숍이나 온라인 과정을 수강합니다.

➢ Reflect on your own biases and ensure they do not influence your care.

자신의 편견을 반성하고 그것이 간호에 영향을 미치지 않도록 합니다.

6. Incorporate Māori Health Models: 마오리 건강 모델 통합

➢ Familiarize yourself with health frameworks like Te Whare Tapa whānau, which includes taha tinana (physical), taha wairua(spiritual), taha whānau(family), and taha hinengaro(mental health).

신체(taha tinana), 정신 건강(taha hinengaro), 가족(taha whānau), 영성(taha wairua)을 포함하는 Te Whare Tapa whānau와 같은 건강 프레임워크를 익힙니다.

➢ Integrate these models into your approach to patient care.

이러한 모델을 환자 간호 접근 방식에 통합합니다.

Common Errors to Avoid

**1. Failure to Respect Cultural Beliefs and Practices
문화적 신념과 관행에 대한 존중 부족**

- Error: Dismissing or not acknowledging Māori cultural values such as mana, wairua, or tikanga.
  * 마오리의 문화적 가치를 무시하거나 인정하지 않음
- Impact: This may cause the patient and whānau (family) to feel disrespected or unsafe, leading to mistrust.
  * 환자와 가족이 존중받지 못하거나 안전하지 않다고 느껴 신뢰를 잃을수 있음
- Solution: Always show respect for and acknowledge cultural beliefs, even if they differ from your own
  * 자신의 신념과 다르더라도 문화적 신념을 존중하고 인정하는 점을 보여줘야 함

2. Poor Communication 의사소통 부족

- Error 1: Using judgmental or dismissive language that undermines the patient's or family's concerns.
  * 환자나 가족의 걱정을 깍아 내리거나 무시하는 판단적인 언어 사용
- Error 2: Speaking in a rushed or overly clinical manner without establishing rapport.
  * 관계를 형성하지 않고 서두르거나 과도하게 임상적인 방식으로 대화함

- Impact: This may create barriers to effective communication and make the patient and whānau feel excluded.
    * 환자와 가족이 배제된 느낌을 주고 이로 인해 효고적인 의사소통에 장벽이 생김
- Solution: Use culturally appropriate greetings such as "Kia ora" or "Tēnā koe." Actively listen and validate the patient's and family's feelings, ensuring clarity and empathy in your communication.
    * 키아오라 또는 테나코에 와 같은 문화적으로 적절한 인사말을 사용하기. 적극적으로 경청하고 환자와 가족의 감정을 공감하며 명확하고 친절한 방식으로 소통하기.

3. Ignoring Family Involvement(Whānau) 가족 참여 무시
- Error: Excluding the family from decision-making or failing to consider their input.
    * 의사결정에서 가족을 배제하거나 의견을 고려하지 않음
- Impact: This can alienate the family and fail to address the collective approach to health that is central to Māori culture.
    * 가족이 소외감을 느끼고 마오리 문화의 핵심인 집단적 건강 접근이 무시될수 있음
- Solution: Actively involve the whānau in discussions, seek their input, and ensure they feel valued as part of the care team.
    * 논의에 가족을 적극적으로 참여시키고 의견을 구하며 그들이 케어팀의 중요한 일부로 존중받는다고 느끼게 하기.

4. Imposing Personal Beliefs or Judgments 개인적 신념 또는 판단 강요

- Error: Imposing personal beliefs onto the patient or family.
  * 환자와 가족에게 자신의 신념을 강요함
- Impact: This can create resistance and reduce the effectiveness of care.
  * 저항을 유발하고 치료 효과가 감소할수 있음
- Solution: Respect the patient's autonomy and decisions, even if they differ from standard medical practices. Advocate for the inclusion of their preferences in the care plan.
  * 표준 의료 관행과 다르더라도 환자의 자율성과 결정을 존중하고, 그들의 선호를 치료계획에 포함하기.

5. Failure to Follow Te Tiriti o Waitangi Principles 테티리티 오 와이탕이 원칙 준수 부족

- Error: Not applying the principles of partnership, protection, and participation in interactions.
  * 협력, 보호 및 참여 원칙을 상호작용에 적용하지 않음
- Impact: This can lead to inequitable care and a lack of cultural safety.
  * 불공평한 케어와 문화적 안전 부족 초래
- Solution: Ensure your care aligns with the Treaty principles:

- Partnership: Work collaboratively with the patient and whānau.
    * 환자와 가족과 협력하기
- Protection: Protect cultural practices and promote equitable healthcare access.
    * 문화적 관행을 보호하고 평등한 의료 접근 촉진
- Participation: Involve the patient and whānau fully in decision-making.
    * 환자와 가족이 의사결정에 완전히 참여하도록 하기

6. Lack of Cultural Knowledge 문화적 지식 부족

- Error: Displaying ignorance about Māori cultural concepts such as Te Whare Tapa Whānau(the Māori health model) or misusing Māori terms.
    * 마오리 건강모델과 같은 마오리 문화 개념에 대한 무지 또는 마오리 용어를 잘못 사용함
- Impact: This can lead to unintentional disrespect or harm to the patient's cultural identity.
    * 무의식적으로 무례할수 상황을 이끌거나 환자의 문화적 정체성을 해칠수 있음.
- Solution: Familiarize yourself with Māori health models and cultural values. Use Māori terms appropriately and with respect.
    * 마오리 건강모델과 문화적 가치를 숙지하기. 마오리 용어를 적절하고 준중있게 사용하기.

📝 예시

- **Patient Name:** Hohepa Tēne, 62-year-old male
- **Diagnosis:** Type 2 diabetes with worsening symptoms requiring hospitalization
- **Cultural Background:** Māori
- **Family:** Spouse, three children, and extended family

The patient has been advised to start insulin therapy for better blood sugar management. However, he states that he cannot make a decision without consulting his family. This reflects the Māori cultural value of **collective decision-making** and **family-centered care**(whānau). As a nurse, your role is to respect the patient's cultural values while facilitating family involvement in decision-making.

· **환자 이름:** Hohepa Tēne(호헤파 타네), 62세 남성
· **진단:** 2형 당뇨병 악화로 인한 입원
· **문화적 배경:** 마오리
· **가족:** 배우자와 3명의 자녀, 가까운 친척 포함

환자는 병원에서 혈당 조절을 위해 인슐린 치료를 권고받았으나, 가족과 논의하기 전에는 결정을 내릴 수 없다고 말합니다. 이는 마오리 문화에서 중요한 **집단적 의사결정**과 **가족 중심적 접근**을 반영한 것입니다. 당신은 간호사로서 환자의 문화를 존중하며 환자와 가족이 참여하는 의사결정을 지원해야 합니다.

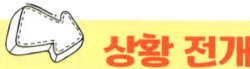 **상황 전개**

1. Initial Contact with the Patient
- **Goal:** Build trust with the patient and understand their cultural needs.
- **Sample Dialogue:**
  - "Tēnā koe, Hohepa.(Hello, Hohepa.) It's a pleasure to work with you. My name is [Name], and I'm your nurse. I understand that your family's involvement is important. Would you like to discuss your treatment options with your whānau(family) before making any decisions?"

2. Acknowledging the Patient's Family Role
- The patient responds, "It's not right for me to make decisions without my whānau."
- The nurse acknowledges this and offers to arrange a family meeting.

---

1. 간호사로서 환자와의 초기 접촉
- **목표:** 환자와 신뢰를 구축하고 문화적 요구를 이해함.
- **대화 예시:**
  - "Tēnā koe, Hohepa.(안녕하세요, 호헤파 씨.) 저와 함께 일하게 되어 반갑습니다. 저는 간호사 [이름]입니다. 치료 과정에서 환자님과 가족의 의견을 중요하게 생각합니다. 혹시 치료 결정을 내리기 전에 가족과 함께 논의하시고 싶으신가요?"

2. 환자와 가족의 중요성 인정하기
- 환자는 "가족 없이 결정을 내리는 것은 우리에게 맞지 않습니다. Whānau(화나우: 가족)가 함께해야 합니다."라고 대답합니다.
- 간호사는 이를 인정하며 가족 회의를 조율합니다.

가족 회의 준비

3. Preparation Steps
- Confirm a convenient time for family members to participate.
- Arrange for a private space where the family feels comfortable.
- Incorporate Māori cultural practices, such as starting the meeting with karakia(prayer), to make the patient and family feel respected.

4. Nurse's Role
- Maintain a neutral and supportive stance while explaining treatment options clearly.
- Allow ample time for the family to discuss and ask questions.

---

3. 실시 전 준비
- 가족이 참여할 수 있는 시간을 확인.
- 프라이버시가 보장되는 공간으로 회의장소 마련.
- 마오리 문화적 요소를 존중하여 환자와 가족이 편안함을 느낄 수 있도록 함.
  예) 가족의 중요성을 상징하는 **카라키아(기도)**로 회의를 시작하도록 제안.

4. 간호사 역할
- 회의에서 중립적인 자세를 유지하며 치료 옵션을 명확히 설명.
- 가족이 질문하고 논의할 시간을 충분히 제공.

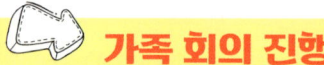 **가족 회의 진행**

5. Starting the Meeting

- "Kia ora, Hohepa's whānau. Thank you for coming. I understand how important your role is in helping Hohepa make decisions about his care. Today, we'll discuss the treatment options and address any questions you may have."
- "Before we begin, would you like to start with karakia(prayer)?"

  (If agreed, a family member leads the karakia.)

6. Explaining Treatment Options

- The nurse explains the treatment plan in simple and clear terms:
  - "At this stage, insulin therapy is recommended to help stabilize Hohepa's blood sugar levels. Let me explain how insulin works, its benefits, and how it can be managed effectively."

---

5. 회의 시작
- "안녕하세요, Hohepa 씨의 가족 여러분. 저는 가족분들이 치료 결정에서 중요한 역할을 한다는 것을 알고 있습니다. 오늘은 Hohepa 씨의 치료 옵션에 대해 함께 논의해 보려고 합니다."
- "회의를 시작하기 전에 카라키아(기도)로 시작하시겠습니까?"
  (가족이 동의하면 카라키아를 진행.)

6. 치료 옵션 설명
- 간호사는 환자와 가족이 이해하기 쉬운 용어를 사용하여 치료 옵션을 설명합니다.
  - "현재 Hohepa 씨의 혈당 조절을 위해 인슐린 치료가 권장되고 있습니다. 이것은 혈당 수치를 안정적으로 유지하는 데 도움이 됩니다. 인슐린 치료의 방법과 기대 효과, 그리고 관리 방법에 대해 자세히 설명드리겠습니다."

7. Providing Time for Family Discussion

- The nurse steps back to allow the family to discuss the information privately.
- During family questions, the nurse responds transparently and respectfully.

8. Supporting the Decision

- After the family discussion, the nurse says, "Take as much time as you need to make a decision. Please let me know if you have any further questions or concerns."

7. 가족 논의 시간 제공
- 간호사는 가족끼리 논의할 시간을 줍니다.
- 가족이 질문할 때 친절하고 투명하게 답변합니다.

8. 결정 지원
- 가족이 논의한 후, 간호사는 "결정을 내리실 때까지 충분한 시간을 드리겠습니다. 언제든 질문이 있으면 저희에게 말씀해주세요."라고 말하며 환자와 가족의 결정을 존중합니다.

Follow-Up Actions

- Share the patient's and family's decision with the healthcare team.
- If the patient agrees, involve the family in follow-up care planning. For instance, provide education on administering insulin or guide the family on how to support the patient with meal planning.
- Continue to encourage family involvement throughout the treatment process.

후속 조치
- 환자와 가족이 결정한 내용을 의료진에게 공유하고, 환자가 원한다면 가족과 함께 후속 치료 계획을 세웁니다.
- 치료 과정 중에도 가족 참여를 지속적으로 장려합니다. 예를 들어, 인슐린 주사 방법을 가족 구성원에게 교육하거나, 식단 관리에 가족이 함께 참여하도록 조언합니다.

Evaluation

- ↳ Ensure the patient and family felt respected and fully involved in the decision-making process.
- ↳ Assess their satisfaction with the treatment plan.
- ↳ Review whether the cultural needs were adequately met during care.

평가
- 환자와 가족이 치료 결정 과정에서 존중받았는지 확인.
- 환자와 가족이 치료 계획에 만족하는지 평가.
- 문화적 요구가 적절히 반영되었는지 검토.

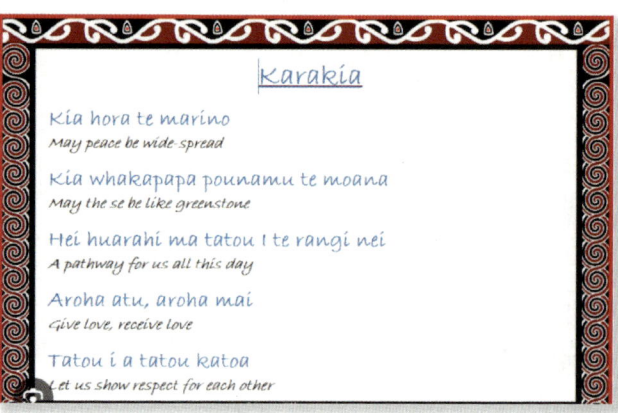

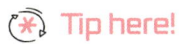
Tip here!

카라키아(Karakia)는 마오리 문화에서 중요한 영적 표현 방식이며 기도 또는 주문을 의미하는 마오리어 용어입니다. 중요한 사건, 의식, 하루의 시작이나 종료 시에 사용되며 신의 축복을 기원하고, 조상이나 자연의 힘에 감사를 표현합니다. 널싱(간호)과 관련하여 카라키아를 적용한다면, 환자와 가족의 마음을 진정시키고, 문화적으로 안전한 간호를 제공하는 데 중요한 역할을 할 수 있습니다.

마킹 기준 체크리스트 Marking Criteria

Category	Step	Met	Not Met
1. Initial patient interaction			
Introduce yourself, your role and patient identity	"Hello, my name is(Name) and I am your nurse today", confirm the Māori patient's details and ensure cultural respect		
Demonstrate awareness of cultural diversity	Acknowledge the significance of cultural identity in healthcare decisions		
Seek to build rapport and trust with the patient	Use open-ended questions and show genuine interest in the patient's well-being		
2. Respecting the patient's autonomy			
Explain the healthcare plan and treatment options clearly	Ensure that the patient fully understands their options in a culturally sensitive manner		
Actively listen to the patient's preferences and values	Demonstrate empathy and active listening		

Respect the patient's decision-making process, including refusal of treatment if applicable	Acknowledge and respect the patient's right to refuse or accept treatment		
3. Family-centred Care			
Involve family in decision-making when appropriate	Engage the family in discussions when the patient desires or cultural protocols require it		
Ensure family members are comfortable and informed	Provide information to family members in a respectful and clear manner		
Ensure the family's wishes are respected in the treatment process	Understand and respect the role of Whānau in decision-making for Māori patients		
4. Cultural Sensitivity			
Acknowledge the importance of spirituality and cultural beliefs in care	Seek to understand and incorporate the patient's cultural and spiritual values in care planning		
Use culturally appropriate language and behaviour	Demonstrate sensitivity to cultural norms and expression when interacting with the patient and family		
5. Clear communication			
Communicate information clearly and respectfully	Use simple, non-technical language and avoid jargon to ensure understanding		
Clarify any doubts and patient or family might have	Ensure that all questions are answered and that the patient and family feel heard		

6. Shared decision-making			
Involve the patient and family in treatment decisions	Demonstrate a collaborative approach to decision-making with the patient and family		
Identify and respect the role of the Māori culture in health decisions	Acknowledge the holistic view of health, including spiritual, physical, and mental well-being		
7. Consent and Documentation			
Obtain informed consent from the patient and /or family	Ensure that informed consent is obtained according to cultural practices and patient understanding		
Accurately document the patient's preferences and decisions	Record all relevant cultural preferences, decisions, and family involvement clearly		
8. Professionalism			
Maintain a respectful and non-judgemental demeanor throughout	Demonstrate cultural humility and professionalism in all interactions.		
Adhere to hospital protocols for cultural competency	Ensure compliance with institutional policies regarding cultural sensitivity and patient-centred care		
Manage time efficiently while ensuring patient and family needs are met	Balance time management with maintaining cultural sensitivity and comprehensive care		

⑤ 응급상황 관리

Station Five: Emergency management
CPR and Automated External Defibrillator (AED) Usage

🔖 스테이션 목표

- 심정지 환자 발생 시 신속하고 효과적인 심폐소생술(CPR)을 수행할 수 있다.
- 자동제세동기(AED)를 안전하고 정확하게 사용하여 환자의 생명을 구할 수 있다.
- DRSABC 접근법을 통해 환자의 상태를 평가하고, 팀워크와 의사소통을 바탕으로 응급 상황을 관리할 수 있다.

🔖 주요 기술

1. DRSABC 접근법 수행:
- Danger: 주변 환경의 위험 확인.
- Response: 환자의 반응 여부 확인(Shake & Shout).
- Send for help: 즉각적으로 응급 상황 알리고 도움 요청.
- Airway: 기도 개방 여부 확인(Head Tilt/Chin Lift).
- Breathing: 환자가 호흡하지 않거나 비정상적 호흡 여부 확인(10초 이내).
- Circulation: 흉부 압박 시행 준비.

2. 심폐소생술(CPR):

- ↝ 흉부 압박:
  - 성인의 경우 흉부를 약 5-6cm 깊이로 누르고 분당 100-120회 속도로 압박.
  - 압박 후 완전히 가슴을 이완시키는 것을 잊지 않기.
- ↝ 인공호흡:
  - 30:2 비율로 흉부 압박과 인공호흡을 반복(일회용 마스크 사용).
  - 인공호흡은 환자의 흉부가 상승하도록 충분히 수행.

3. 제세동기(AED) 사용:

- ↝ AED를 환자 곁에 준비하고 전원을 켬.
- ↝ 패드를 환자의 가슴에 올바르게 부착(오른쪽 쇄골 아래, 왼쪽 옆구리).
- ↝ AED가 "Analysing" 상태에서 **"Stand Clear"**를 외쳐 모든 사람이 환자에게서 떨어지도록 함.
- ↝ AED가 제세동(Shock)을 권장하면, **"Stand Clear"**를 재확인한 뒤 충격 버튼을 누름.
- ↝ 이후 즉각적으로 CPR 재개.

4. 환자와 주변 상황 모니터링:

- ↝ CPR과 AED 사용 중 환자의 상태와 주변 환경을 지속적으로 관찰.

🔖 평가 기준

1. **DRSABC 수행 여부**: 응급 상황 초기 평가와 도움 요청이 적절하게 이루어졌는지 확인.
2. **심폐소생술 기술**: 흉부 압박과 인공호흡이 올바른 비율과 깊이/속도로 이루어졌는지 평가.
3. **제세동기 사용**: AED 패드 부착과 지시에 따른 충격 수행 여부 평가.
4. **의사소통 및 팀워크**: 상황을 명확히 전달하고, 주변 사람들과 협력하며 지시를 내릴 수 있는 능력 평가.
5. **시간 관리**: 제한된 시간 내에 필요한 응급 처치를 신속하게 수행했는지 평가.
6. **감염 관리**: 손 위생과 PPE 사용 여부 확인(상황과 가능여부에 따라 다를수 있음).

🔖 학습 팁

1. **DRSABC 숙달**: CPR을 시작하기 전 DRSABC 과정을 체계적으로 연습하세요.
2. **압박 기술 연습**: 흉부 압박은 정확한 깊이와 속도가 중요하므로, 마네킹을 사용해 지속적으로 연습하세요.
3. **AED 사용법 숙지**: AED의 사용 지침과 패드 부착 위치를 정확히 익혀야 합니다.
4. **팀워크 시뮬레이션**: 다른 학습자들과 팀을 구성해 CPR과 AED 사용 중 의사소통과 역할 분담을 연습하세요.
5. **실제 상황 가정**: 긴급 상황에서도 침착하게 수행할 수 있도록 다양한 시나리오로 연습하세요.
6. **시간 관리**: 제한된 시간 내에 모든 절차를 완료할 수 있도록 연습하며 속도와 정확성을 동시에 신경 쓰세요.
7. **체계적 마무리**: CPR과 AED 절차 후 환자의 상태를 계속 모니터링하며 도움 요청 상태를 확인하세요.

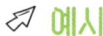 예시

1. Preparation: 준비

↳ Ensure the scene is safe for both the rescuer and the patient.

구조자와 환자 모두에게 현장이 안전한지 확인합니다.

↳ Gently shake the patient's shoulders and ask loudly, "Are you okay?" to check for responsiveness.

환자의 어깨를 부드럽게 흔들며 큰 소리로 "괜찮으세요?"라고 물어보며 반응이 없는지 확인합니다.

↳ Please avoid using a sternum rub to assess responsiveness, as it is considered an outdated practice.

반응을 확인하기 위해 흉골 마찰법(스턴럼 러브)을 사용하지 마십시오. 이는 현재 권장되지 않는 practice입니다.

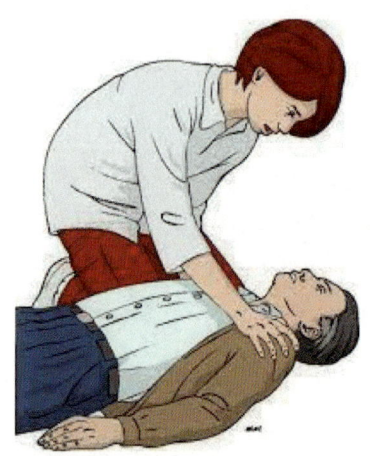

- Call for help: "Someone call emergency services and bring the AED."

> 도움 요청: "누군가 응급 서비스를 호출하고 AED를 가져오세요."
> (뉴질랜드 emergency response number is 111 입니다.)

- Check the Airway , Breathing; head tilt and chin lift, look listen and feel, no more than 10 second – If the patient is unresponsive and not breathing normally, begin the CPR immediately.

> 환자가 반응이 없고 정상적으로 숨을 쉬지 않는 경우 즉시 심폐소생술을 시작합니다.

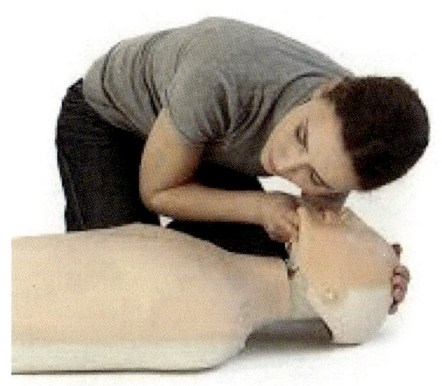

 Tip here!

> 심폐소생술과 제세동기 사용에 대한 스테이션에서 무엇보다 기억해야 할 점은 DRSABC입니다.

First AID CPR

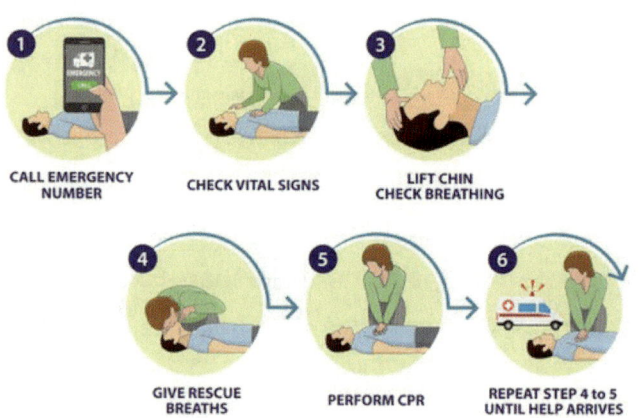

2. Step-by-Step Procedure for CPR: 심폐소생술 단계별 절차

2.1 Positioning: 위치

- Ensure the patient is lying flat on a firm surface(e.g., the floor).

환자가 단단한 바닥(예: 바닥)에 평평하게 누워 있는지 확인합니다.

- Kneel beside the patient at chest level.

환자의 가슴 높이에 무릎을 꿇고 앉습니다.

2.2 Chest Compressions: 흉부압박

- Place the palm of one hand on the center of the patient's chest(lower half of the sternum).

한 손의 손바닥을 환자의 가슴 중앙(흉골 하부)에 놓습니다.

- Place the other hand on top and interlock your fingers.

다른 손을 위에 올리고 손가락을 깍지 낍니다.

- Keep your arms straight, position your shoulders directly over your hands, and compress firmly and quickly.

팔을 곧게 펴고 어깨를 손 바로 위에 위치시키며 강하고 빠르게 압박합니다.

- Perform compressions at a rate of 100-120 per minute and a depth of at least 5 cm(2 inches) but no more than 6 cm(2.4 inches).

분당 100~120회의 속도로, 깊이는 최소 5cm(2인치)에서 최대 6cm(2.4인치)까지 압박합니다.

- Allow the chest to fully recoil between compressions while keeping your hands in contact with the chest.

흉부압박 사이에 흉부가 완전히 되돌아가도록 시간을 주며 손은 가슴에 계속 닿아 있어야 합니다.

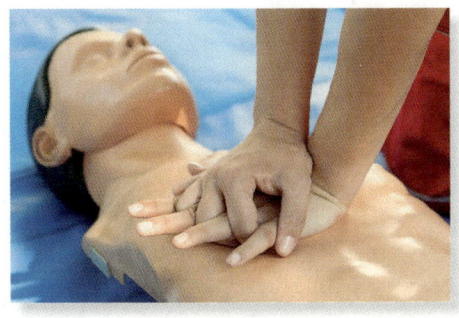

2.3 Rescue Breaths 구조호흡

✒ After 30 chest compressions, tilt the head back and lift the chin to open the airway.

30회의 가슴 압박 후 턱을 들어 올려 기도를 확보합니다.

✒ Pinch the patient's nose and cover their mouth with yours to give two breaths.

환자의 코를 막고 자신의 입으로 밀폐하여 2번 숨을 불어넣습니다.

✒ Each breath should last about 1 second, ensuring the chest visibly rises.

각 호흡은 약 1초 정도 지속되어야 하며 가슴이 눈에 띄게 올라야 합니다.

✒ Resume chest compressions immediately after giving breaths.

호흡 후 즉시 가슴 압박을 재개합니다.

✒ Continue alternating 30 compressions with 2 breaths.

30회의 압박과 2회의 호흡을 반복합니다.

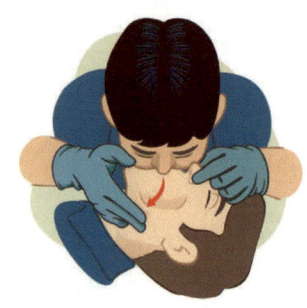

3. Using the AED: AED 사용

3.1 Turn on the AED: AED 켜기

↳ Open the AED and press the power button to turn it on.

AED를 열고 전원 버튼을 눌러 켭니다.

↳ Follow the device's voice prompts.

기기의 음성안내를 따릅니다.

3.2 Attach the Pads: 패드부착

↳ Expose the patient's chest and ensure it is dry.

환자의 가슴을 드러내고 건조한지 확인합니다.

↳ Ensure the bystander continues CPR while the AED pads are being attached.

제세동기 패스 부착시 bystander가 심폐소생술을 계속 지속하도록 합니다.

↳ Attach the adhesive pads to the patient's chest as indicated by the diagrams on the pads:

패드에 표시된 그림에 따라 접착 패드를 환자의 가슴에 부착합니다.

- Place one pad below the right collarbone. 오른쪽 쇄골아래
- Place the other pad on the lower left side of the chest, 왼쪽 겨드랑이 아래

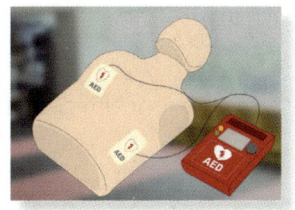

3.3 Rhythm Analysis: 리듬분석

- After attaching the pads, ensure no one is touching the patient.(also make sure pads are not touching the clothes)

패드를 부착한 후 누구도 환자에게 닿지 않도록 합니다.(또한 패드가 옷에 닿지 않도록 합니다.)

- Press the "Analyze" button if necessary(depending on the AED model, analysis may occur automatically). When analysing, all need to be clear.(make sure to say-stand clear!)

필요하면 "분석" 버튼을 누릅니다(AED 종류에 따라 자동으로 분석하기도 합니다). 분석시 누구도 환자를 터치 하지 않아야 합니다.

- Follow the AED's instructions.

AED의 지침을 따릅니다.

3.4 Delivering a Shock(if recommended): 충격 제공(권장될 경우)

- If the AED recommends a shock, ensure no one touches the patient.

AED가 충격을 권장하면 환자에게 아무도 닿지 않았는지 확인합니다.

- Loudly announce, "Stand Clear!" and visually confirm that no one is in contact with the patient.

큰 소리로 "비켜주세요!"라고 외치고 아무도 환자에게 닿지 않았는지 시각적으로 확인합니다.

⤳ Press the shock button to deliver the shock.

충격 버튼을 눌러 충격을 제공합니다.

 Tip here!

제세동기가 Analysing을 할때 Stay clear를 외쳤더라도, 제세동기가 shock을 권장하면 다시한번 stay clear를 외쳐 누구도 환자에게 닿지 않는것을 확인합니다.

4. Resume CPR: 심폐소생술 재개

⤳ Immediately resume chest compressions after delivering the shock.

즉시 가슴 압박부터 CPR을 재개합니다.

⤳ Continue to follow the AED's instructions.

AED의 지침을 계속 따릅니다.

5. Repeat if Necessary: 필요시 반복

⤳ Continue performing CPR and following the AED's instructions until emergency services arrive or the patient shows signs of life, such as movement or normal breathing.

CPR을 계속 시행하고 AED 지침을 따르며, 응급 서비스가 도착하거나 환자가 움직임이나 정상적인 호흡과 같은 생명 신호를 보일 때까지 진행합니다.

6. If need to handover paramedics or medical staff

➢ Use the ISBAR handover tool-introduce yourself, provide details about the patient if known, hand over information on how many cycles of CPR have been performed and how many AED shocks have been delivered. Recommend transferring the patient to the emergency department(ED) for post-CPR care or appropriate medical care.

> ISBAR 인수인계 도구를 사용하세요. 본인을 소개하고 환자에 대해 알고 있는 정보를 제공하며, 수행된 CPR 사이클 수와 AED 충격 횟수를 전달합니다. 환자를 응급실(ED)로 이송하여 CPR 후 치료 또는 적절한 의료 처치를 받을 것을 권장합니다.

 Tip here!

ISBAR은 의료진 간의 효과적인 의사소통을 위한 구조화된 프레임워크입니다. 이는 환자 상태 변화나 악화 시 정보를 명확하고 간결하게 전달하는 데 특히 유용합니다. ISBAR의 각 요소는 다음과 같습니다.

I - 신원 확인
- 자신과 상대방의 신원을 명확히 합니다.
- 본인의 이름, 직책, 소속을 밝힙니다.

S - 상황 설명
- 환자의 기본 정보(이름, 나이, 성별 등)를 제공합니다.
- 현재 환자의 상태나 문제를 간단히 설명합니다.

B - 배경 정보
- 환자의 주요 증상과 관련 병력을 요약합니다.
- 현 상황에 관련된 중요한 정보를 공유합니다.

A - 평가
- 환자의 활력징후를 포함한 현재 상태를 평가합니다.
- 비정상적인 징후나 우려사항을 강조합니다.

R - 권고사항
- 필요한 조치나 처치를 제안합니다.
- 조치의 긴급성과 시기를 명시합니다.

이 프레임워크를 사용하면 의료진 간 의사소통이 더욱 체계적이고 효율적으로 이루어질 수 있습니다. 이는 결과적으로 환자 안전과 케어의 질 향상으로 이어집니다.

Common Mistakes to Avoid

1. Failing to check for unresponsiveness and abnormal breathing before starting CPR.
   * 심폐소생술을 시작하기 전에 무반응 및 비정상적인 호흡을 확인하지 않음.
2. Performing shallow or slow chest compressions.
   * 얕거나 느린 가슴 압박 수행.
3. Interrupting chest compressions unnecessarily and putting the hands in the wrong place
   * 가슴 압박을 중단하거나 손을 잘못된 위치에 두는 경우
4. Incorrectly attaching the AED pads.
   * AED 패드의 부적절한 부착.
5. Failing to confirm everyone is clear before delivering a shock.
   * 충격을 제공하기 전에 모두가 비켰는지 확인하지 않음.

마킹 기준 체크리스트 Marking Criteria

Category	Step	Met	Not Met
1. Initial Assessment			
Ensure the scene is safe	Confirms the environment is safe for rescuer and victim, remove hazards		
Check for responsiveness	Tap the victim and shout " Are you Okay?"		
Call for help	Shout for assistance and ensure someone calls emergency services(e.g. : 111) and retrieve an AED		
Check breathing	Perform a head tilt, chin lift and looks, listens, and feels for normal breathing for 5-10 seconds		
Identify cardiac arrest and start CPR	Confirm the patient is unresponsive and not breathing and start chest compression within 2 mins		
2. Chest Compressions			
Position hands correctly	Place the heel of one hand in the centre of the chest(lower half of the sternum) and interlocks fingers		
Deliver compressions at proper depth	Compress the chest to a depth of 5-6cm(2-2.4 inches) for adults		
Deliver compressions at proper rate	Maintain a rate of 100-120 compressions per minute		

Allows full chest recoil	Ensure the chest completely recoils after each compression		
3. Rescue Breaths			
Provide effective rescue breaths	Deliver two breaths using a pocket mask, ensuring visible chest rise		
Maintain proper technique	Ensure a proper seal and reposition if chest does not rise		
Alternate compressions and breaths	Provide a 30:2 compression-to breath ratio		
4. AED Usage			
Turn on the AED	Powers on the AED immediately upon its arrival		
Attach AED pads correctly-	Place pads as per AED instructions(e.g. upper right chest and lower left side of the chest)		
Ensure no contact during analysis	State "Stand clear!" and confirm no one is touching the patient during rhythm analysis		
Deliver shock if advised	Press the shock button after AED prompt and ensure safety by confirming no contact		
Resume compressions promptly	Immediately resume chest compressions after shock delivery		
5. Post CPR Reassessment			
Check for signs of life	Assess for breathing, movement or other signs of life periodically between cycles		

Prepare for handover to paramedics or Medical team member	Provide a concise handover to emergency responders, detailing interventions performed and patient status(e.g. ISBAR framework)		
6. Professionalism			
Communicate effectively	Maintain clear and professional communication with team member or bystanders		
Demonstrate confidence	Appear calm, focused, and in control throughout the scenario		
Manage time efficiently	Complete all actions promptly and within a reasonable time frame		

6 임상 술기(상처드레싱 교환)

Station Six: Clinical skills
Change the wound dressing (ANTT) & TIME assessment

🏁 스테이션 목표

- 환자의 상처를 평가하고 TIME 사정 도구를 활용해 상처 상태를 체계적으로 분석할 수 있다.
- 무균적 기법(Aseptic Non touch Technique : ANTT)을 적용해 상처 드레싱을 안전하고 효과적으로 교환할 수 있다.
- 환자와 소통하며 상처 관리와 관련된 교육을 제공하고, 환자의 안전과 감염 예방을 보장한다.

🏁 주요 기술

1. 상처 평가와 TIME 사정:
- **T(Tissue):** 괴사조직(죽은 조직) 또는 육아조직(건강한 조직)의 유무를 평가.
- **I(Infection/Inflammation):** 감염 징후(발적, 분비물, 열감, 통증 등) 또는 염증 여부를 확인.
- **M(Moisture):** 상처가 지나치게 건조하거나 과도한 삼출물이 있는지 평가.
- **E(Edge):** 상처 가장자리 상태를 확인(들떠 있거나 상처가 좁혀지는지 관찰).

2. 무균적 기법(Aseptic Technique):
- 손 위생을 철저히 수행하고, 필요한 PPE(장갑, 가운 등)를 착용.
- 깨끗한 드레싱 장비를 준비하고 소독제를 사용하여 상처 부위를 세척.
- 드레싱 교환 과정 동안 무균 상태를 유지하며 오염 방지.

3. 드레싱 교환:
- 기존의 드레싱을 제거하며, 제거된 드레싱의 상태(냄새, 색, 삼출물 양 등)를 관찰.
- 상처 부위를 멸균 생리식염수로 세척하고, 감염 위험이 있는 부위를 주의 깊게 소독.
- 새로운 드레싱을 상처 상태에 맞게 적용하며, 부착 후 상태를 확인.

4. 환자와의 소통:
- 환자에게 드레싱 교환 과정을 설명하고, 불편감을 최소화하기 위해 배려.
- 환자에게 상처 관리와 감염 예방 교육을 제공(예: 손 위생, 드레싱 유지 방법).

⚘ 평가 기준

1. **TIME 사정의 적절성**: 상처의 조직 상태, 감염 여부, 삼출물, 가장자리 등을 체계적으로 평가했는지 확인.
2. **무균적 기법의 적용**: 드레싱 교환 과정에서 무균 상태를 유지하고 감염 예방 원칙을 준수했는지 평가.
3. **드레싱 교환의 정확성**: 적절한 도구와 기술을 사용하여 드레싱을 안전하게 교환했는지 확인.
4. **환자 안전 및 편안함**: 환자의 불편감을 최소화하며, 안전하게 상처 관리가 이루어졌는지 평가.

5. **의사소통 능력**: 환자와 명확하고 친절한 소통을 통해 신뢰를 구축하고 교육을 효과적으로 제공했는지 확인.
6. **시간 관리**: 제한된 시간 내에 드레싱 교환과 상처 사정을 효과적으로 수행했는지 평가.

🔖 학습 팁

1. **TIME 사정 연습**: TIME 도구를 활용해 상처 상태를 분석하는 연습을 반복하세요. 다양한 사례를 통해 실력을 키우는 것이 중요합니다.
2. **무균 기법 습득**: 드레싱 교환 시 무균 상태를 유지하는 과정을 반복적으로 연습하며 감염 예방 기술을 숙달하세요.
3. **드레싱 종류 숙지**: 다양한 상처에 적합한 드레싱 재료와 사용법을 미리 학습하세요.
4. **환자 중심의 접근**: 환자와의 소통 능력을 키우고, 상처 관리 중 환자의 불편감을 최소화하는 방법을 고민하세요.
5. **사례 기반 학습**: 실제 시나리오와 유사한 상황에서 TIME 사정과 드레싱 교환을 수행하며 실전 감각을 익히세요.

🔖 예시

1. Preparation and Infection Control 준비 및 감염관리

➢ Perform hand hygiene using soap and water or an alcohol-based hand sanitizer.

> 비누와 물 또는 알코올 기반 손 소독제를 사용하여 손 위생을 수행합니다.

➢ Assemble all necessary equipment, including gloves, dressing pack, saline, and waste disposal bag.

> 장갑, 드레싱 키트, 생리식염수, 폐기물 처리 봉투 등 필요한 모든 장비를 준비합니다.

- Explain the procedure to the patient: "I'll be changing your wound dressing to promote healing and prevent infection. Do you have any questions before we begin?"

> 환자에게 절차를 설명합니다: "상처 드레싱을 교체하여 치유를 촉진하고 감염을 예방하려고 합니다. 절차를 시작하기 전에 질문이 있으신가요?"

- Ensure patient privacy and position them comfortably, exposing only the wound area.

> 환자의 프라이버시를 보장하고, 상처 부위만 노출되도록 환자를 편안하게 위치시킵니다.

2. TIME Framework Overview:

- The TIME framework guides wound assessment and management:
  - **T:** Tissue viability
  - **I:** Infection or inflammation
  - **M:** Moisture balance
  - **E:** Edge of the wound

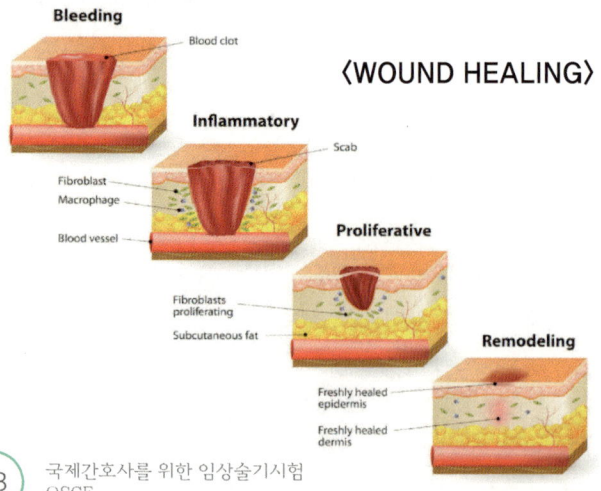

〈WOUND HEALING〉

3. Procedure Steps

3.1 Remove the Old Dressing: 기존 드레싱 제거

↠ Don non-sterile gloves and carefully remove the old dressing.

> 비멸균 장갑을 착용하고 기존 드레싱을 조심스럽게 제거합니다.

↠ Observe the old dressing for any signs of infection (e.g., odor, discharge) and discard it in a clinical waste bag.

> 기존 드레싱에서 감염징후(예: 냄새, 분비물) 을 관찰하고 폐기물 봉투에 폐기합니다.

↠ Perform hand hygiene after removing gloves.
장갑을 제거한 후 손 위생을 수행합니다.

3.2 Assess the Wound(TIME Framework): 상처평가

↠ Tissue Viability: 조직 생존력
  - Look for healthy granulation tissue(red and moist) or necrotic tissue(black, yellow, or brown) and document it

> 건강한 육아 조직(빨갛고 촉촉한 조직) 또는 괴사 조직(검은색, 노란색, 갈색)을 확인하고 기록 합니다.

↠ Infection or Inflammation: 감염 또는 염증
  - Check for redness, swelling, warmth, or excessive exudate.

> 발적, 부기, 온기 또는 과도한 삼출물을 확인합니다.

- Note any foul odor or increased pain, which may indicate infection.

> 악취 또는 통증 증가와 같은 감염 징후를 기록합니다.

- ↳ Moisture Balance: 수분 균형
  - Assess for excess fluid or dryness. A moist environment promotes healing, but excessive moisture can cause maceration.

> 과도한 수분 또는 건조 여부를 평가합니다. 촉촉한 환경은 치유를 촉진하지만, 과도한 수분은 피부 연화를 초래할 수 있습니다.

- ↳ Edge of the Wound: 상처 가장자리
  - Observe if the edges are attached or undermined. Rolled or detached edges may indicate delayed healing.

> 가장자리가 부착되어 있는지 또는 분리되어 있는지 관찰합니다. 말려 올라가거나 분리된 가장자리는 치유 지연을 나타낼 수 있습니다.

3.3 Clean the Wound: 상처 세척

- ↳ Prepare the sterile field
  - Open the dressing pack using Aseptic non-touch technique(ANTT)to ensure sterility
  - Avoid touching any sterile items with unsterile hands or surfaces.

- 무균 비접촉 기술(ANTT)을 사용하여 드레싱 키트를 열어 멸균 상태를 유지한다.
- 멸균 물품을 비멸균 손이나 표면과 접촉하지 않도록 주의한다.

↳ Don sterile gloves.
- Use saline or the prescribed solution to clean the wound, ensuring that the sterile gauze and solution are handled using non-touch technique.

생리 식염수 또는 처방된 용액을 사용하여 상처를 세척하며, 비접촉 기술을 사용하여 멸균 거즈와 용액을 다룬다.

- Clean the wound starting from the center and moving outward in a circular motion, taking care not to touch the wound directly.

상처 중심에서 외곽으로 원을 그리고 닦고, 상처를 직접적으로 만지지 않도록 주의한다.

↳ Prevent cross-contamination
- Use separate sterile gauze for each wipe to maintain sterility and prevent cross-contamination.

닦을 때마다 별도의 멸균 거즈를 사용하여 멸균 상태를 유지하고 교차감염을 방지한다.

- Dispose of used gauze and materials into the appropriate waste container immediately, ensuring sterile items remain untouched.

사용한 거즈와 재료는 즉시 적절한 폐기물 용기에 버리며, 멸균 물품이 오염되지 않도록 한다.

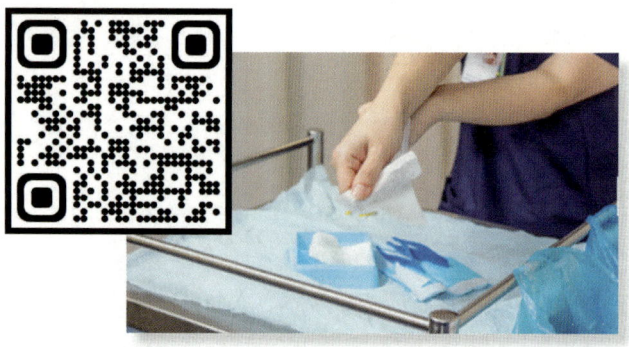

3.4 Apply the New Dressing: 새 드레싱

⤻ Ensure the wound is dry before applying the new dressing.

새 드레싱을 적용하기 전에 상처를 건조하게 유지합니다.

⤻ Select an appropriate dressing based on the TIME assessment

TIME사정에 따라 적절한 드레싱을 선택합니다.

- For a dry wound, use a hydrogel dressing to maintain moisture.

건조한 상처의 경우, 수분을 유지하기 위해 하이드로겔 드레싱을 사용합니다.

- For an exudative wound, use an absorbent dressing.

삼출물이 많은 상처의 경우, 흡수 드레싱을 사용합니다.

- Secure the dressing with adhesive tape or bandages without causing tension on the skin.

> 피부에 긴장이 가지 않도록 접착 테이프나 붕대로 드레싱을 고정합니다.

3.5 Dispose of Waste and Perform Hand Hygiene: 폐기물 처리 및 손 위생 수행

- Discard all used materials in a clinical waste bag.

> 사용한 모든 물품을 의료 폐기물 봉투에 폐기합니다.

- Remove gloves and perform hand hygiene.

> 장갑을 제거하고 손 위생을 수행합니다.

4. Closing the Procedure:

4.1 Patient Education and Comfort: 환자 교육 및 편안함 제공

- Inform the patient about the wound's condition and any signs of infection to watch for: "The wound is healing well, but please let us know if you notice increased redness, swelling, or discharge."

> 상처 상태와 감염 징후에 대해 환자에게 설명합니다: "상처는 잘 치유되고 있습니다. 하지만 발적, 부기 또는 분비물이 증가하면 알려주세요."

- Reposition the patient for comfort and ensure their dignity is maintained.

> 환자를 편안한 자세로 재배치하고 존엄성을 유지합니다.

4.2 Documentation:

↳ Record the wound assessment(using the TIME framework), the dressing used, and the patient's response to the procedure.

상처 평가(TIME 프레임워크 사용), 사용된 드레싱 및 절차에 대한 환자의 반응을 기록합니다.

Common Errors to Avoid

1. Failing to maintain aseptic technique, leading to contamination.
   * 무균 기술을 유지하지 않아 그것이 오염을 유발할수 있는 행위
2. Neglecting a thorough TIME assessment, which may result in improper wound management.
   * 철저한 TIME 평가를 소홀히 하여 부적절한 상처 관리로 이어짐.
3. Applying a dressing that is inappropriate for the wound's moisture level.
   * 상처의 수분 수준에 적합하지 않은 드레싱을 적용함.
4. Not documenting key observations and actions.
   * 주요 관찰 및 조치를 문서화하지 않음.

📋 마킹 기준 체크리스트 Marking Criteria

Category	Step	Met	Not Met
1. Preparation			
Review patient's care plan and wound history	Confirm the type, location, and care instructions for the wound		
Gather necessary equipment	Collect dressing pack, gloves, cleaning solution, and waste disposal bag		
Perform hand hygiene	Wash hands according to WHO standars before starting the procedure		
Ensure the environment is clean and safe	Prepare a clean and private workspace		
2. Patient preparation			
Introduce yourself and explain the procedure	Gain informed consent and ensure patient understanding		
Position the patient comfortably	Ensure the wound site is accessible while maintaining patient's dignity		
3. Dressing Removal			
Perform hand hygiene and don gloves	Use appropriate personal protective equipment(PPE)		
Remove the old dressing safely	Use aseptic technique to avoid contamination		
Dispose of the old dressing appropriately	Place the used dressing in a clinical waste bag immediately		

4. TIME Assessment			
T - Tissue: Assess the wound bed for tissue type	Identify granulation, slough, or necrotic tissue and document findings		
I - Infection/Inflammation: identify signs of infection	Observe for redness, swelling, heat, exudate, or odor		
M - Moisture: Evaluate moisture balance	Note if the wound is too dry or excessively moist		
Edge: Inspect wound edges	Assess for undermining, maceration, or healthy edge migration		
5. Wound Cleaning			
Use ANTT and Clean the wound under guidelines	Use prescribed cleaning solution and work from the cleanest to dirtiest area		
Avoid contamination during cleaning	Ensure no cross-contamination occurs during the process		
6. Dressing Application			
Apply the appropriate dressing	Select and secure a dressing suitable for the wound type and condition		
Ensure the dressing is secured properly	Confirm that the dressing is fixed without causing discomfort		
7. Post-Procedure care			
Remove gloves and perform hand hygiene	Follow correct procedure for glove removal and sanitization		

Reposition the patient and ensure comfort	Make sure the patient is comfortable, and the wound site is protected		
8. Documentation			
Document wound assessment findings	Record TIME findings and any abnormalities noted		
Document the dressing change procedure	Include date, time, dressing type and patient response		
9. Professionalism			
Communicate effectively with the patient	Ensure clear and empathetic communication throughout the procedure		
Adhere to infection control protocols	Maintain aseptic technique and PPE usage consistently		
Manage time efficiently	Complete the procedure within the allocated time		

❼ 약물 투약

Station Seven: Medication Administration

📌 스테이션 목표

- 환자에게 안전하고 정확한 방법으로 약물을 투여할 수 있다.
- 약물 계산을 정확히 할수 있다.
- 약물의 효과, 부작용, 그리고 환자의 상태를 고려하여 투여 전, 중, 후 과정을 철저히 관리한다.
- 약물 투여 시 7가지 권리(7 Rights)를 준수하며, 간호사로서의 책임감을 가지고 약물 관리 프로세스를 수행한다.
- 환자와의 소통을 통해 약물 관련 정보를 제공하고, 환자의 질문이나 우려 사항을 해결한다.

📌 주요 기술

1. 약물 투여 전 확인

- 7가지 권리(7 Rights):
  - 올바른 환자, 약물, 용량, 시간, 경로, 목적, 기록을 확인.
- 환자 정보(이름, 생년월일)를 확인하고, 알레르기 여부를 물어본다.
- 약물 처방과 약물 라벨을 두 번 이상 확인하며, 필요한 경우 동료 간호사와 크로스체크한다.
- 정확한 약물 계산을 실행한다.

- 약물 투여 목적과 적응증을 이해하고, 환자의 현재 상태(예: 혈압, 혈당, 통증 등)를 평가한다.

2. 약물 준비와 투여 과정
- 무균 기법을 유지하며 약물을 준비.
- 적절한 투여 경로(경구, 근육 주사, 정맥 주사 등)에 따라 약물을 투여.
- 투여 과정 중 환자에게 설명하며, 편안함을 제공.

3. 약물 투여 후 관리
- 투여 후 환자의 반응과 부작용 여부를 관찰.
- 필요 시, 추가 평가(예: 통증 감소 여부, 혈압 변화 등)를 수행.
- 환자에게 약물의 효과와 복용 방법, 부작용 발생 시 대처 방법을 교육.

4. 문서 작성
- 투여한 약물 이름, 용량, 경로, 시간, 반응 등을 정확히 기록.
- 약물 투여와 관련된 모든 사항을 병원 프로토콜에 맞게 문서화.

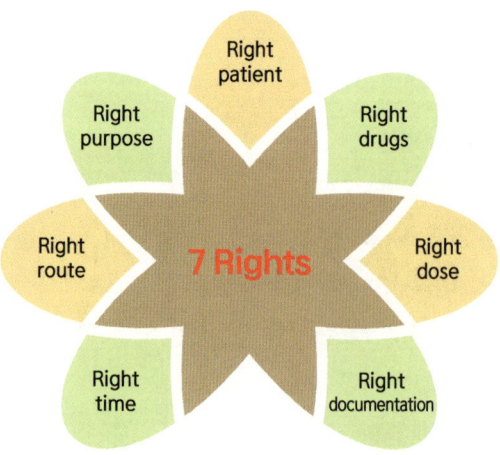

평가 기준

1. 7가지 권리 준수 여부:
- 약물 투여 전, 중, 후에 7 Rights를 철저히 지켰는지 평가.

2. 투여 기술의 정확성:
- 무균 기법과 투여 과정에서의 기술적 능력을 평가.
- 투여 경로에 맞는 올바른 절차를 따랐는지 확인.

3. 환자와의 소통 능력:
- 환자에게 투여 과정과 약물 정보를 명확하고 이해하기 쉽게 전달했는지 평가.
- 환자의 질문이나 우려를 효과적으로 해결했는지 확인.

4. 안전성:
- 알레르기 여부, 약물 상호작용, 환자의 상태를 고려했는지 평가.
- 약물 부작용 및 투여 후 반응 관찰 여부를 확인.

5. 시간 관리:
- 제한된 시간 내에 정확하고 신속하게 약물 투여 과정을 수행했는지 평가.

6. 문서 작성의 완성도:
- 투여 기록이 정확하고, 병원 프로토콜에 맞게 작성되었는지 확인.

Tip here!

뉴질랜드에는 약물투여와 관련된 두가지 책이 항상 병동에 구비되어 있습니다. IV관련 책은 NOIDS라고 하고 Oral 관련 책은 MIMS라고 합니다.

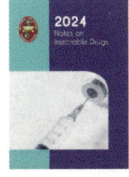
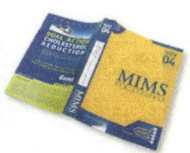

NOIDS(National Online Interactive Drug Information System)
NOIDs는 주사제(Injectable Drugs)에 대한 정보를 제공하는 전문 참고 자료입니다. 약물의 안정성, 혼합 가능성, 희석 방법, 투여 경로, 저장 조건 등을 포함하여 주사제의 안전한 사용을 위한 세부 정보를 제공합니다. 간호사나 약사가 주사제를 준비하거나 투여할 때 약물의 혼합과 관리가 안전하게 이루어질 수 있도록 돕는 데 사용됩니다. 특히, 약물 간 상호작용과 안정성에 중점을 둡니다.

MIMS(Monthly Index of Medical Specialties)
약물에 대한 정보를 정리한 포괄적인 참고 자료로, 종이책 및 디지털 형식으로 제공됩니다. 약물의 성분, 작용 메커니즘, 용량, 적응증, 부작용 등을 쉽게 찾아볼 수 있도록 구성되어 있습니다. 다양한 약물 정보를 신속하게 찾아보고, 처방과 약물 관리에 활용됩니다.
이 두 자료는 의료 실무에서 중요한 참고 자료로, 약물 안전성과 환자 치료를 위한 정확한 정보를 제공합니다.

학습 팁

1. 7가지 권리 숙지:
↳ 약물 투여의 기본 원칙인 7 Rights를 철저히 이해하고, 매번 실습에서 이를 반복적으로 확인하세요.

2. 약물 지식 강화:
↳ 시험에서 자주 등장하는 약물의 용량, 효과, 부작용 등을 미리 학습하세요.

3. 투여 기술 연습:
↳ 경구 약물, 근육 주사(IM), 피하 주사(SC), 정맥 주사(IV) 등 경로별로 기술을 반복 연습하세요.

4. 환자 중심 소통:
↳ 환자에게 약물 정보를 전달하고, 질문에 답하는 시뮬레이션 연습을 통해 소통 능력을 강화하세요.

5. 시간 관리:
↝ 시험 시간 안에 모든 절차를 완료하는 연습을 하세요. 각 단계별로 소요 시간을 줄이는 방법을 고민하세요.

6. 시뮬레이션 활용:
↝ 모의 환자를 활용하여 실제와 같은 환경에서 약물 투여 과정을 연습하세요.

예시

1. Preparation and Infection Control:
↝ Perform hand hygiene using soap and water or an alcohol-based hand sanitizer.

> 비누와 물 또는 알코올 기반 손 소독제를 사용하여 손 위생을 수행합니다.

↝ Verify the patient's identity using two identifiers(e.g., name, date of birth) and also check national health index(NHI) number & **Allergies.**

> 환자의 이름, 생년월일을 확인하고 또한 NHI number와 알러지를 확인합니다.

↝ Check the medication chart and prescription for accuracy and completeness. Ensure the five rights of medication administration are adhered to

> 환자의 약물챠트와 처방전을 확인합니다. 약물 투여의 7가지 원칙을 준수합니다.

- Right patient 올바른 환자
- Right medication 올바른 약물
- Right dose 올바른 용량
- Right route 올바른 경로
- Right time 올바른 시간
- Right purpose 올바른 목적
- Right documentation 올바른 기록

➢ Explain the procedure to the patient: "I'm here to administer your medication. I'll explain what it is for and ensure it's given correctly. Do you have any questions?"

환자에게 절차를 설명합니다: "지금 약물을 투여하려고 합니다. 약물의 용도를 설명드리고 정확하게 투여도록 하겠습니다. 질문이 있으신가요?"

2. Procedure Steps:

2.1 Verify and Prepare the Medication: 약물 확인 및 준비

➢ Cross-check the medication name, dose, route, and time on the prescription with the medication chart.

처방전의 약물 이름, 용량, 경로 및 시간을 약물 차트와 교차 확인합니다.

➢ Inspect the medication for expiration dates and any visible abnormalities.

약물의 유효 기간과 눈에 띄는 이상 여부를 검사합니다.

➢ Prepare the medication using aseptic techniques. For oral medications, pour the correct dose into a clean medication cup. For injectable medications, draw up the prescribed dose into a sterile syringe.

무균 기술을 사용하여 약물을 준비합니다. 경구 약물의 경우, 올바른 용량을 깨끗한 약물 컵에 따릅니다. 주사 약물의 경우, 처방된 용량을 멸균 주사기에 준비합니다.

➢ If required, calculate the correct dose and double-check your calculations with a colleague.

필요한 경우, **올바른 용량을 계산**하고 동료와 함께 계산을 재확인합니다.

Tip here!

한국도 같은 시스템이겠지만 뉴질랜드는 특히 더블체크를 아주 중시 합니다. IV로 들어가는 모든 약과 controlled drugs(규제약물, 예를 들어 Morphine, Fentanyl, Codeine, tramadol 등)과 아동 16세 미만에게 주어지는 약은 꼭 동료와 함께 더블체크하고 싸인을 함께 해야 합니다.

2.2 Confirm Patient Understanding and Consent: 환자 이해 및 동의 확인

➢ Explain the purpose of the medication and potential side effects to the patient: for example, "This medication is to lower your blood pressure. You might feel slightly dizzy at first, but that's normal."

약물의 목적과 잠재적인 부작용을 환자에게 설명합니다: 예를 들어 "이 약물은 혈압을 낮추기 위한 것입니다. 처음에는 약간 어지러움을 느낄 수 있지만 이는 정상입니다."

↪ Confirm if the patient has any allergies or previous adverse reactions to the medication.

환자가 약물에 대한 알레르기나 이전에 부작용을 경험한 적이 있는지 확인합니다.

2.3 Administer the Medication: 약물투여
↪ For oral medications: 경구약물
- Offer the patient a glass of water.

환자에게 물 한잔을 제공합니다.

- Observe as they swallow the medication to ensure compliance.

환자가 약물을 삼키는 것을 관찰하여 복약 순응도를 확인합니다.

↪ For injectable medications: 주사 약물
- Choose the correct injection site

올바른 주사 부위 선택

- Clean the site with an alcohol swab and allow it to dry.

알코올 솜으로 부위를 닦고 건조시킵니다.

- Administer the injection at the correct angle(e.g., 90° for intramuscular, 45° for subcutaneous).

올바른 각도로 주사를 투여합니다.(예: 근육주사는 90°, 피하주사는 45°).

2.4 Post-Administration Monitoring: 투여후 모니터링

↪ Observe the patient for any immediate adverse reactions or side effects.

> 즉각적인 부작용이나 이상 반응이 있는지 환자를 관찰합니다.

↪ Provide reassurance and ensure they are comfortable: "Please let me know if you feel any discomfort or unusual symptoms."

> 환자에게 안심을 주고 편안함을 보장합니다: "불편함이나 이상 증상이 있으면 알려주세요."

2.5 Patient Education: 환자 교육

↪ Provide the patient with information about the medication, including its purpose, how it works, and any potential side effects.

> 약물의 목적, 작용 원리 및 잠재적인 부작용에 대한 정보를 환자에게 제공합니다.

↪ Encourage them to ask questions or voice concerns about their medication regimen.

> 약물 요법에 대한 질문이나 우려 사항을 제기하도록 환자를 격려합니다.

↪ Educate the patient on signs of adverse reactions to watch for and when to seek medical attention.

> 부작용의 징후를 확인하고 의료 조치가 필요한 경우를 교육합니다.

2.6 Documentation 기록

↪ Record the medication name, dose, route, time, and any observations in the patient's chart.

↪ If the patient refused the medication, document the reason and inform the healthcare team.

- 약물 이름, 용량, 경로, 시간 및 관찰 사항을 환자의 차트에 기록합니다.
- 환자가 약물을 거부한 경우, 이유를 문서화하고 의료팀에 알립니다.

Common Errors to Avoid

1. Failing to verify patient identity, leading to potential administration errors.
   * 환자의 신원을 확인하지 않아 발생할 수 있는 투여 오류.
2. Administering medication without confirming allergies or contraindications.
   * 알레르기나 금기사항을 확인하지 않고 약물을 투여하는 것.
3. Errors in medication administration by ensuring accurate dosage calculations.
   * 약물 용량 계산을 정확히 하지 않아 생기는 오류
4. Skipping documentation, which may result in incomplete records and potential safety issues.
   * 문서화를 생략하여 기록이 제대로 마무리 되지 않고 안전 문제가 발생하는 경우
5. Using incorrect techniques for injectable medications, causing discomfort or complications.
   * 부정확한 기술을 사용하여 불편함이나 합병증을 유발하는 것.

마킹 기준 체크리스트 Marking Criteria

Category	Step	Met	Not Met
1. Preparation			
Review patient's prescription and medication chart	Verify correct patient, medication, dose, route, timing and purpose(7Rs)		
Check for allergies or contraindications	Confirm any documented allergies and cross-checks with the patient		
Gather necessary equipment	Prepare the required medication, syringe, water, gloves etc		
Ensure a clean and safe environment	Prepare a sterile and organised workspace		
2. Patient Identification and Consent			
Confirm patient identity using two identifiers	Verify name, Date of Birth(DOB) or hospital number		
Explain the procedure and gain consent	Ensure the patient understands and agrees to the administration		
Provide an opportunity for the patient to ask questions	Encourage patient engagement and address any concerns		
3. Medication preparation			
Check the medication label against theh prescription	Ensure the medication is correct andnot expired		
Calculate the correct dose if required	Demonstrate accurate dose calculation		

Prepare the medication using aseptic technique	Ensure no contamination during preparation		
4. Administration process			
Perform hand hygiene and don gloves if necessary	Follow infection control protocols		
Recheck the medication and patient detail before administration	Ensure correct medication is administrared to the right patient		
Administer the medication via the correct route	Oral, IV, subcutaneous etc using proper technique		
Monitor the patient during administration	Observe for any immediate adverse reactions		
5. Post administration Care			
Ensure the patient is comfortable and safe	Reassure the patient and monitor for delayed reactions		
Dispose of used equipment appropriately	Follow waste disposal and sharp handling protocols		
6. Documentation			
Accurately record the medication administered	Include drug name, dose, route, time, purpose and signature		
Document any patient response or adverse events	Note any unusual reactions or patient feedback		

9. Professionalism			
Maintain a professional demeanor throughout	Demonstrate confidence, respect, and empathy		
Adhere to safety protocols and policies	Ensure compliance with institutional and national guidelines		
Manage time efficiently	Complete the procedure within the allocated time		

8 의사소통 및 팀워크

Station Eight: Communication and teamwork

🏷 스테이션 목표

1. Effective Delegation 효과적인 업무분배
↪ Manage the acute situation by assigning roles and responsibilities to team members.
급성상황을 관리하며 팀원들에게 역할과 책임을 배정한다.

2. Prioritization 우선순위 설정
↪ Ensure urgent care is provided to the deteriorating patient while routine tasks are delegated appropriately.
긴급한 환자케어가 제공되도록 하고 루틴 작업은 적절히 위임한다.

3. Clear and Collaborative Communication 명확하고 협력적인 의사소통
↪ Foster teamwork and ensure all team members are clear on their tasks and responsibilities.
팀워크를 강화하고 모든 팀원이 자신의 업무와 책임을 명확히 이해하도록 한다.

4. Maintaining Professionalism 전문성 유지

- Remain calm and composed, especially during stressful situations, to lead the team effectively.
  스트레스가 많은 상황에서도 침착하고 차분하게 행동하여 팀을 효과적으로 이끈다.

주요기술

1. Clinical Prioritization 임상적 우선순위 설정

- Recognize and address the urgent care required for the deteriorating patient.
  악화된 환자에게 필요한 긴급케어를 인지하고 처리한다.
- Delegate routine care tasks to other team members.
  루틴케어 작업을 다른 팀원에게 위임한다.

2. Delegation with Clarity

- Assign tasks using concise, step-by-step instructions.
  명확한 업무분배, 간결하고 단계별로 이해하기 쉬운 지시를 제공한다.

3. ISBAR Communication Framework ISBAR의사소통 프레임 워크

- Use the ISBAR framework to convey patient information clearly and efficiently to team members.
  환자 정보를 명확하고 효율적으로 팀원들에게 전달한다.

4. Team Coordination 팀조정

- Ensure all team members are aware of the plan and can report back if issues arise.
  모든 팀원이 계획을 이해하고 문제가 발생할 경우 보고 할수 있도록 한다.

✱ Tip here!

뉴질랜드 간호에서 Direction(지도)과 Delegation(위임)은 환자 안전과 의료팀의 효율성을 보장하기 위해 매우 중요한 개념입니다. 간단히 설명드리면,

1. Direction(지도)
간호사가 팀 내 다른 의료 종사자(예: 보조 간호사 또는 간호 지원 인력)에게 업무를 수행하도록 지시하고, 이를 지속적으로 감독하는 과정입니다. 이는 업무가 적절하게 수행되고 있는지 확인하여 환자 안전을 보장하고 팀 구성원이 각자의 역할을 명확히 이해하고 책임을 다할 수 있도록 지원하는데 큰 의미를 둡니다. 이는 또한 환자 상태의 변화에 신속히 대응할 수 있도록 큰 의미를 지닙니다.

2. Delegation(위임)
간호사가 특정 업무를 적절한 훈련과 자격을 가진 다른 의료 종사자에게 위임하는 과정입니다.
업무를 위임함으로써 간호사는 더 복잡하고 전문적인 간호에 집중할 수 있고 팀의 효율성을 높이고 환자에게 더 나은 서비스를 제공할수 있습니다. 위임된 업무는 항상 간호사의 감독과 책임 하에 이루어져야 하며, 위임전에는 항상 위임받는 사람의 역량과 환자 요구 사항을 고려해야 합니다.
뉴질랜드 간호에서 지도와 위임은 환자 중심 케어를 제공하고 의료팀의 협력과 신뢰를 증진시키는 데 핵심적인 역할을 합니다. 간호사는 최종 책임을 지는 위치에 있기 때문에, 지도와 위임 과정에서 정확성과 책임감이 필수적입니다.

⌕ 평가기준

1. Leadership: 리더쉽
↳ Demonstrates confidence and assertiveness in leading the team.
팀을 이끄는데 있어 자신감과 단호함을 보여준다.

2. Prioritization: 우선순위 설정
↳ Addresses the deteriorating patient as a priority while ensuring other patients' needs are not neglected.
악화된 환자를 우선적으로 관리하며 다른 환자의 요구가 무시되지 않도록 보장한다.

3. Clarity of Communication: 의사소통 명확성
↝ Provides detailed, easy-to-understand instructions to team members.
팀원들에게 상세하고 이해하기 쉬운 지시를 제공한다.

4. Teamwork and Collaboration: 팀워크와 협력
↝ Engages team members respectfully and collaborates effectively to achieve goals.
팀원들을 존중하며 효과적으로 협력한다.

5. Follow-Up:
↝ Checks in with team members to monitor progress and reassess priorities.
팀원들에게 작업진행 상황을 확인하고 우선순위를 재평가한다.

⌲ 학습팁

1. Practice Acute Scenarios: 급성 상황 연습
↝ Simulate situations involving deteriorating patients and practice delegating tasks while maintaining patient safety.
악화된 환자를 다루는 상황을 시뮬레이션하고 환자 안전을 유지하며 업무를 분배하는 연습을 한다.

2. Learn ISBAR: ISBAR학습
↝ Practice using the SBAR framework for communicating with team members or escalating to doctors.
팀원에게 업무를 전달하거나 의사에게 상황을 보고할때 ISBAR프레임워크를 사용하는 연습을 한다.

3. Time Management: 시간관리
↳ Focus on making decisions quickly and assigning tasks efficiently to avoid delays in care.
결정을 빠르게 내리고 업무를 효율적으로 할당하여 케어지연을 방지한다.

4. Team Awareness: 팀 역량 이해
↳ Know the roles and skills of your team members to assign tasks effectively.
팀원들의 역할과 기술을 파악하여 업무를 효과적으로 분배한다.

5. Follow-Up: 후속 확인
↳ After delegating tasks, always check back with team members to ensure tasks are completed and identify any issues.
업무를 위임한 후 항상 팀원들에게 진행 상황을 확인하고 문제가 없는지 확인한다.

예시

You notice that Mr. John Smith(Room 2) is in respiratory distress with SpO$_2$ at 85%. You act quickly to assign tasks to your team of three:

> 당신원 2번방의 John Smith씨가 산소 포화도가 85%로 떨어지며 호흡곤란을 겪고 있는 것을 발견했습니다. 즉시 다음과 같이 팀원들에게 업무를 할당합니다.

You(Team Leader): 팀 리더

↳ **(To Nurse A):**

"Nurse A, Mr. John Smith in Room 2 is in respiratory distress. Please assess his airway, ensure his oxygen is connected and set to 15L via non-rebreather mask. Take his vital signs and prepare to escalate if needed. Let me know his response to oxygen therapy."

> 간호사 A, 2번방의 John Smith씨가 호흡곤란을 겪고 있어요. 그의 기도를 확인하고 산소마스크를 15L로 연결해 주세요, 그의 활력징후를 측정하고 산소 요법에 대한 반응을 관찰하고, 필요시 상황이 악화되시 보고할 준비를 해주세요. 산소요법에 반응이 있는지 알려주세요.

↳ **(To Nurse B):**

"Nurse B, while Nurse A is stabilizing Mr. Smith, can you please change the wound dressing for Mrs. Green in Room 3. Ensure sterile technique and assess the wound for signs of infection. Let me know if there's anything concerning."

> 간호사 B, 간호사 A가 Smith씨를 안정화하는동안 3번방의 Green씨의 상처 드레싱을 교체해 주세요. 무균기술을 사용하고 감염징후가 있는지 평가해 주세요. 문제가 있으면 보고해 주세요.

↳ **(To Healthcare Assistant):**

"Sarah, please assist Mr. Brown in room 4 to the bathroom. He has mobility difficulties, so make sure to support him carefully. Pay close attention to fall prevention while assisting him. Let me know once he is safely back in bed or if there are any issues."

> Sarah, 4번 방의 Brown 씨를 화장실에 데려다 주세요. 거동이 불편하시니 꼭 조심히 부축해 주세요. 도와드리는 동안 낙상 예방에 특히 신경 써 주세요. 무사히 침대로 돌아오시면 알려주시고, 문제가 생기면 바로 보고해 주세요.

↳ (To the Team):

"Team, let's meet back here in 15 minutes for a quick update. I'll monitor Mr. Smith's response to the oxygen therapy and be available for assistance if needed."

> 팀, 15분 후에 다시 만나 업데이트를 논의합시다. 저는 Smith 씨의 산소 치료 반응을 모니터링하며 필요 시 도움을 줄 수 있도록 대기하겠습니다.

Common Errors to Avoid

1. **Failure to Prioritize: 우선순위 설정 실패**
   - Neglecting the deteriorating patient to focus on routine tasks.
   * 상태가 악화되는 환자를 무시하고 루틴 작업에 집중하는 것
2. **Unclear Instructions: 불명확한 지시**
   - Providing vague or incomplete directions that confuse team members.
   * 모호하거나 불안전한 지시로 인해 팀원들이 혼란을 겪음
3. **Overloading One Team Member: 한명에게 과도한 업무 부여**
   - Assigning multiple tasks to one person without considering their workload.
   * 한 사람에게 여러 작업을 과중하게 할당하는 것

4. **Ignoring Follow-Up**: 업무 분할후에 확인하지 않는것
   - Not checking back with team members to ensure tasks are completed effectively.
   * 팀원들이 업무를 제대로 해내는지 확인하지 않는것

5. **Lack of Calmness**: 부족한 침착한 자세
   - Appearing stressed or unorganized, which can undermine team confidence.
   * 스트레스를 받고 조직적이지 않은 모습을 보여 팀 신뢰를 저하시키는 것

🖋 마킹 기준 체크리스트 Marking Criteria

Category	Step	Met	Not Met
1. Initial Preparation			
Ensure a clear understanding of the task at hand	Demonstrate awareness of patient needs and priorities		
Review the skills and competencies of team members	Consider the qualifications and scope of practice of colleagues before delegating		
2. Clear communication			
Clearly define the task to be delegated	Provide a specific and concise description of the task		
Communicate expected outcomes and deadlines	Ensure the team member understands the goals and timeline for task completion		
Use respectful and professional language	Demonstrate effective interpersonal communication skills		

3. Assigning tasks			
Assign tasks based on team member's competencies and workloads	Match the task to the appropriate team member's skill level and capacity		
Provide necessary instructions and clarify doubts	Ensure team members have all the required information to perform the task		
Encourage team members to ask questions or seek clarification	Create an open and supportive communication environment		
4. Monitoring and follow-up			
Regularly check on the progress of the delegated task	Provide oversight without micromanaging		
Offer support and assistance when needed	Ensure team members feel supported while performing their tasks		
Acknowledge and address any challenge encountered	Take action to resolve issues in a timely manner		
5. Feedback and recognition			
Provide constructive feedback on task performance	Highlight strengths and areas for improvement		
Recognise and appreciate team member's contributions	Express gratitude and reinforce positive teamwork		

6. Conflict resolution(If needed)			
Identify and address any team conflicts promptly	Maintain a collaborative and harmonious team environment		
Mediate disagreements professionally	Demonstrate fair and unbiased conflict resolution skills		
9. Professionalism			
Demonstrate leadership and accountability	Lead the team effectively and take responsibility for the outcomes		
Maintain a calm and composed demeanor	Ensure effective communication under pressure		
Adhere to hospital protocols and scope of practice	Ensure all tasks are assigned within the legal and professional framework		

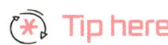
 Tip here!

뉴질랜드의 EWS 시스템(Early Warning System)은 병원 및 의료 환경에서 환자의 상태 변화를 조기에 감지하고, 적절한 조치를 취할 수 있도록 돕는 체계입니다. 이 시스템은 환자의 활력 징후(Vital Signs)를 점수화하여 임상적인 악화를 조기에 예측하고 관리하는 데 사용됩니다. 아래는 뉴질랜드 EWS 시스템의 주요 특징입니다:

〈예시〉

Vital Signs		Date	17/6/17
		Time (24 hour)	18:24
Respiratory Rate (breaths/min) write **RR** value in box		≥ 36	
		25-35	**34**
		21-24	
		12-20	
		9-11	
		5-8	
		≤ 4	
Oxygen (L/min)		Room air ✓	
		Supplement (L/min)	**2**
Oxygen Saturation (%) write **SpO₂** value in box		≥ 96	**96**
		94-95	
		92-93	
		≤ 91	
Heart Rate (bpm) mark **HR** with X write value if off scale		Write if ≥ 140	
		130s	
		120s	
		110s	
		100s	
		90s	
		80s	X
		70s	
		60s	
		50s	
		40s	
		30s	

Blood Pressure (mmHg) score systolic **BP** value only	Write if ≥ 220	
	210s	
	200s	
	190s	
	180s	
	170s	
	160s	
	150s	
	140s	
	130s	
	120s	
	110s	
	100s	
	90s	
	80s	
	70s	
	60s	
	50s	
Temperature (°C) mark **Temp** with X write value if off scale	≥ 39s	
	38s	
	37s	X
	36s	
	35s	
	≤ 34s	
Level Of Consciousness mark **LOC** with ✓	Alert	✓
	Voice	
	Pain	
	Unresponsive	
EARLY WARNING SCORE TOTAL		**5**

1. EWS의 목적
- 환자의 **상태 변화**를 조기에 발견합니다.
- 악화된 환자에 대해 **안전하고 신속하며 효과적인 관리**를 제공합니다.
- 환자의 생체 징후를 점수화하여, 환자의 상태를 쉽게 평가하고 즉각적인 조치를 결정할 수 있습니다.

2. EWS 사용이 중요한 이유
- **임상적 판단을 보조:** EWS는 간호사와 의료진의 임상 평가를 지원하여 더 나은 결정을 내릴 수 있도록 돕습니다.
- **의사소통 도구:** 환자를 다른 부서로 이동하거나 임상적 지원을 요청할 때, EWS 점수를 기반으로 환자의 상태를 정확하게 전달할 수 있습니다.
- **모든 환자에게 적용:** 병원 내 모든 환자에게 생체 징후를 기록할 때 반드시 EWS를 사용하여 상태 변화를 모니터링해야 합니다.

3. EWS 활용 방법
1) 생체 징후 관찰 및 기록:
- 환자의 호흡수, 심박수, 혈압, 체온, 산소포화도, 의식 수준 등을 확인하여 점수를 계산합니다.
- 점수가 높을수록 환자의 상태가 더 위험하다는 것을 의미합니다.

2) 변화 감지:
- 점수 변화가 있으면 이를 즉시 확인하고, 환자가 더 악화되기 전에 필요한 조치를 취합니다.

3) 환자 이동 시 의사소통:
- 환자를 다른 부서로 옮기거나 의사의 도움을 요청할 때 EWS 점수를 함께 전달합니다.
- 정기적으로 EWS를 계산하지 않는 전문 부서에서도 환자 이동 시에는 반드시 EWS 점수를 계산해야 합니다.

4. EWS 도구
- 병원에서 사용하는 생체 징후 기록 차트에는 EWS 계산을 위한 도구가 포함되어 있습니다.
- 점수 계산이 자동화되어 있거나 차트에서 손쉽게 확인할 수 있도록 설계되어 있습니다.

5. 핵심 메시지
- EWS는 간호사가 환자의 상태 변화를 놓치지 않도록 돕는 필수적인 도구입니다.
- 이를 통해 환자의 안전을 강화하고, 치료 효과를 극대화할 수 있습니다.
- 모든 간호사가 EWS를 올바르게 사용하면, 팀 간 협력과 환자 관리의 품질을 높일 수 있습니다.

이처럼 EWS는 간단하지만 매우 중요한 시스템입니다. 이를 숙지하고 활용하면 환자의 생명을 구하는 데 큰 기여를 할 수 있습니다.

⑨ 간호계획 수립

Station nine: Planning nursing care

🏹 스테이션 목표

이 스테이션의 주요 목표는 간호사가 임상적 추론을 적용하고 환자 중심의 간호 계획을 수립할 수 있는 능력을 평가하는 것입니다. 핵심적인 문제를 식별하고, 실현 가능한 목표를 설정하며, 증거 기반의 중재를 설계하는 능력이 중요합니다. 간호사는 환자의 필요를 고려하여 우선순위를 정하고, 정확하게 문서화하는 능력을 보여야 합니다.

🏹 주요 기술

환자 정보 분석 및 우선순위 결정: 간호사는 환자의 병력, 현재 상태, 활력 징후 등 관련 정보를 분석하여 가장 중요한 문제를 식별하고 우선순위를 정해야 합니다. 긴급한 문제와 덜 중요한 문제를 구별하여 적절한 순서로 간호를 제공할 수 있어야 합니다.

- **간호 문제 식별:** 간호사는 환자의 상태를 바탕으로 최소 두 가지 주요 간호 문제 또는 요구를 식별해야 합니다. 이 문제들은 환자의 병력과 현재 증상에 부합해야 합니다.
- **적절한 간호 목표 설정:** 식별된 간호 문제를 바탕으로 명확하고, 측정 가능하며, 실현 가능한 목표를 설정해야 합니다. 목표는 환자

중심적이어야 하며, 지정된 시간 내에 달성 가능한 것이어야 합니다.
- **증거 기반 간호 중재 계획:** 간호사는 최신 연구와 모범 사례 지침을 바탕으로 간호 중재를 계획해야 합니다. 이러한 중재는 식별된 간호 문제를 해결하고, 필요에 따라 약물적 및 비약물적 접근을 포함해야 합니다.
- **정확한 간호 기록 작성:** 간호 계획은 명확하고 간결하게 문서화되어야 하며, 간호사는 식별된 간호 문제, 목표, 중재 및 평가 방법을 정확한 의학 용어로 기록해야 합니다. 기록은 읽기 쉽고 법적 기준을 충족해야 합니다.

평가 기준

- **명확하고 읽기 쉬운 필체로 답변 작성:** 간호 계획은 명확하게 작성되거나 타이핑되어야 하며, 다른 의료 전문가들이 쉽게 읽고 이해할 수 있도록 구조화되어야 합니다.
- **두 가지 관련 간호 문제/요구 식별:** 간호사는 환자의 건강 상태와 임상적 증상을 바탕으로 최소 두 가지 주요 간호 문제나 요구를 정확하게 식별해야 합니다.
- **두 문제에 대한 목표 설정:** 식별된 각 문제에 대해 명확하고 측정 가능한 목표를 설정해야 하며, 목표는 실현 가능하고 현실적이어야 합니다.
- **적절한 평가 날짜 설정:** 평가 날짜는 현실적이어야 하며, 적절한 후속 조치를 위한 기회를 제공해야 합니다. 이 날짜는 간호 문제의 긴급성에 맞춰 설정되어야 합니다.
- **증거 기반 간호 중재 계획:** 간호 중재는 최신의 증거 기반 실천, 모범 사례 및 관련 임상 지침을 반영해야 합니다.
- **전문 용어 사용:** 간호사는 전문적인 간호 언어를 사용하고, 약어나 두문자어는 피해야 합니다. 약어는 임상 환경에서 공통적으로

사용되는 경우만 허용됩니다.
- **오류 수정 시 가독성 유지:** 간호 계획에서 오류가 발생할 경우, 수정은 읽기 쉽게 하고 전체적인 가독성을 유지해야 합니다.
- **정확한 서명 및 날짜 기입:** 간호 계획에 정확한 서명과 날짜를 기입해야 하며, 이는 평가 및 실행을 위해 적절하게 준비되어야 합니다.
- **전문적 행동 준수:** 간호사는 NMC(2018)의 '간호사, 조산사 및 간호보조사의 전문적 실무 및 행동 기준'에 맞춰 전문적인 행동을 보여야 합니다. 이는 윤리적 원칙, 환자 비밀 보장, 환자 중심의 간호 접근 방식을 포함합니다.

학습 팁:

- **APIE 프레임워크(A: 평가, P: 계획, I: 실행, E: 평가)에 익숙해지세요:** APIE 프레임워크는 간호 계획을 구조화하는 데 필수적입니다. 이 프레임워크를 사용하여 모든 환자 간호 측면을 논리적으로 다룰 수 있도록 연습하세요.
- **시간 관리 연습:** 주어진 제한 시간 내에 간호 계획을 완성해야 합니다(보통 14분). 시간을 효과적으로 관리하여 두 가지 주요 문제를 다룰 수 있도록 연습하세요.
- **환자 중심 간호 계획:** 간호 중재를 계획할 때, 환자의 개별 상황을 고려해야 합니다. 예를 들어, 환자의 신체 능력, 병에 대한 이해도, 지원 시스템, 감각 장애 등을 고려하세요.
- **다양한 측면을 간호 계획에 통합하세요:** 간호 계획에는 문화적 안전성, 감염 관리, 대인 커뮤니케이션 전략 등 다양한 측면을 포함해야 합니다.
- **정확한 의학 용어 사용:** 간호 계획을 작성할 때 정확한 의학 용어를 사용하고, 약어는 피하세요. 약어 사용은 임상 환경에서 일반적으로 사용되는 경우에만 허용됩니다.

- **평가 기준 숙지:** 평가 기준을 숙지하고 각 항목을 충족시키는 연습을 하세요. 각 항목을 만족시키는 방법에 대해 미리 연습하여 실수를 줄이세요.
- **임상적 추론 연습:** 우선순위 문제와 중재 결정을 내릴 때 임상적 추론을 적용하세요. 환자의 상태를 이해하고, 계획된 중재가 가져올 결과를 예측하는 연습을 하세요.

예시

Situation: A 65-year-old male patient is two days post-operative after a right hip replacement surgery. He is experiencing pain and expressing anxiety related to movement and mobility. The nurse needs to develop a nursing care plan for this patient.

Task: Develop a comprehensive nursing care plan addressing the patient's pain management and mobility concerns.

> 65세 남성 환자가 우측 고관절 전치환술 후 2일째입니다. 환자는 통증을 호소하고 있으며, 움직임에 대한 불안감을 표현하고 있습니다. 간호사는 이 환자를 위한 간호 계획을 수립해야 합니다.
> 과제: 이 환자를 위한 간호 계획을 수립하되, 통증 관리와 이동 문제를 중심으로 계획을 작성하세요.

Patient Information:
- **Age:** 65 years old
- **Gender:** Male
- **Procedure:** Right hip replacement surgery (2 days post-op)
- **Presenting Issues:** Pain and anxiety related to movement

Nursing Problems/Needs: 간호문제/필요

1. Acute Pain related to right hip replacement surgery, as evidenced by the patient's complaint of pain and discomfort.

> 급성통증 : 우측 고관절 전치환술과 관련된 통증, 환자가 통증을 호소하고 불편함을 느끼는 것과 관련.

2. Impaired Physical Mobility related to surgery and pain, as evidenced by the patient expressing anxiety about movement and limited movement capabilities.

> 신체 보행 능력 저하: 수술 및 통증과 관련하여 환자가 거동에 불안감을 느끼고 보행하는 것에 제한이 있는것과 관련.

Nursing Goals:

1. Pain Management Goal: 통증 관리
↝ The patient will report a decrease in pain to a tolerable level(less than 4/10 on the pain scale) by the end of the shift, within the next 12 hours.

> 환자가 통증강도가 총 10점 중 4점 이하로 감소했다고 보고한다.(통증 척도 기준)

↝ The patient will demonstrate the use of pain management techniques to control discomfort(e.g., deep breathing, repositioning, use of prescribed analgesics).

환자가 통증 완화를 위한 기법(예를 들어 깊은 호흡, 자세 변경, 처방된 진통제 사용)을 활용할수 있다.

2. Mobility Goal:

↪ The patient will demonstrate increased confidence in movement(able to move with assistance) within 24 hours.

환자가 24시간 내에 최소한의 도움으로 보행에 자신감을 보인다.

↪ The patient will be able to participate in daily activities (e.g., sitting up in bed, standing, or transferring from bed to chair) with minimal assistance within 48 hours.

환자가 48시간 내에 최소한의 지원으로 일상적인 활동(예를 들어 침대에서 일어나 앉기, 침대에서 의자까지 이동하기)에 참여할수 있다.

 Interventions:

1. Pain Management: 통증관리

↪ Administer prescribed analgesics(e.g., opioids, non-steroidal anti-inflammatory drugs) as per the patient's pain level and in line with the prescribed schedule.

처방된 진통제(예를 들어 진통제, 항스테로이드 항염제)를 환자의 통증 수준에 맞춰 주기적으로 투여한다.

- Encourage the use of non-pharmacological pain relief measures(e.g., guided imagery, relaxation techniques, and deep breathing exercises).

비약물적 통증 완화 방법(예를 들어 심상 훈련, 이완기겁, 깊은 호흡) 을 사용하도록 격려한다.

- Reassess pain every 2 hours to ensure adequate pain control.

통증을 2시간 마다 재평가하여 통증이 적절히 관리되고 있는지 확인한다.

- Provide a calm and comfortable environment, minimizing noise and light disturbances, to help reduce the patient's anxiety.

환자가 편안하게 휴식할수 있도록 조용하고 어두운 환경을 제공하여 불안을 최소화한다.

- Offer education on the importance of reporting pain early to prevent it from becoming more severe.

통증이 심해지기 전에 미리 통증을 보고할수 있도록 교육한다.

2. Mobility:

- Assist with early mobilization by helping the patient sit up in bed, dangle legs over the side, and gradually progress to standing with assistance.

환자가 침대에 앉을 수 있도록 하고 침대 옆으로 다리를 내려 서는 연습을 도와주도록 한다.

↣ Encourage and assist with passive range of motion exercises for the right leg to improve circulation and prevent joint stiffness.

우측 고관절 수동운동을 격려하여 혈액순환을 개선하고 관절 경직을 예방한다.

↣ Provide a walker or crutches for support and assist the patient in using them properly when moving.

환자가 보행기나 목발로 보행할때 제대로 사용할수 있도록 돕는다.

↣ Educate the patient about safety measures during mobility, such as avoiding twisting or bending the affected hip to prevent injury.

보행중 지켜야 할 안전 사항, 예를 들어 수술한 쪽 관절을 비틀거나 구부리는 동작등을 하지 않도록 주의시킨다.

↣ Monitor vital signs before and after mobilization to ensure there are no complications(e.g., orthostatic hypotension).

보행 전후로 활력징후를 모니터링하여 이상징후가 없는지 살핀다.

3. Psychological Support:

↣ Offer reassurance and listen actively to the patient's concerns about movement and recovery.

환자가 보행에 대한 불안감을 표현할 경우, 적극적으로 경청하고 위로한다.

↳ Encourage the patient to express any fears or anxieties about their mobility and help them develop a plan to address these concerns.

환자가 보행에 대해 두려움을 느끼는 부분을 이야기 하도록 격려하고, 이를 해결할 수 있는 방법을 함께 고민한다.

↳ Provide education on the expected recovery process and how early mobilization is beneficial to healing.

회복 과정과 초기 보행이 회복에 중요하다는 교육을 제공한다.

4. Education:

↳ Teach the patient about the importance of pain management, proper use of mobility aids, and the need to gradually increase mobility as they recover.

통증관리방법, 보행 보조 기구 사용법, 그리고 점진적 보행증진에 대한 교육을 실시한다.

↳ Reinforce the importance of follow-up care for pain management and physical therapy.

통증관리에 대한 후속 케어와 물리치료의 중요성을 강조하고 이를 통해 더 빠르고 안전한 회복이 가능하다는 점을 설명한다.

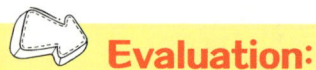

Evaluation:

1. Pain Management:
- Evaluate if the patient reports a pain level of less than 4/10 by the end of the shift.
- Determine whether the patient is using pain management strategies effectively and has less anxiety about the pain.

2. Mobility:
- Assess the patient's ability to safely participate in activities such as sitting up, standing, and transferring with minimal assistance.
- Observe the patient's confidence and ability to move with mobility aids.

마킹 기준 체크리스트 Marking Criteria

Category	Step	Met	Not Met
1. initial patient assessment			
Perform hand hygiene and don gloves if required	Follow infection control protocols		
Confirm patient identity and introduce yourself	Demonstrate respect and clear communication		
Assess the patient's vital signs and pain levels	Measure BP, pulse, respiratory rate, oxygen saturation, temperature accurately and pain score		
Assess the surgical site for any signs of infection or complications	Check for redness, swelling or drainage		
Note the patient's concerns about movement and pain	Acknowledge patient's anxiety and address it empathetically		
2. Pain management			
Review the pain management plan and ensure it's in place	Verify prescribed mendications, routes and timing		
Administer prescribed analgesia and reassess pain level	Provide medication as per orders and reassess the patient's pain score		
Educate the patient on the importance of pain control and how to report discomfort	Provide clear instructions to the patient regarding pain management		

3. Mobility and positioning			
Discuss with the patient their concerns regarding mobility	Validate patient's fear of movement and address it appropriately		
Assist the patient with safe mobilisation using appropriate equipment	Demonstrate proper transfer techniques with walking frame or assistance		
Provide guidance on weight-bearing restrictions and positioning	Educate the patient on the correct positioning to prevent dislocation		
Instruct the patient on leg positioning and use of pillows to maintain hip precautions	Correctly advise on keeping the operated leg in a neutral position		
4. Psychological support			
Offer reassurance and emotional support to reduce anxiety	Demonstrate empathy, actively listening to patient's concerns		
Explain the surgical process and recovery expectations	Provide clear and honest information regarding recovery timelines		
5. Preventing complications			
Assess for signs of deep vein thrombosis(DVT) and encourage mobility	Monitor for signs of swelling, redness, or tenderness in legs		

Encourage coughing and deep breathing exercise to prevent Post op respiratory complications	Demonstrate the importance of respiratory exercises to the patient		
Monitor for signs of infection at the surgical site	Check for increased redness, temperature or drainage at the incision site		
6. Education and Discharge planning			
Educate the patient on the rehabilitation process and follow-up care	Discuss the next steps in therapy and rehabilitation		
Ensure the patient understands discharge instructions, including wound care and follow-up appointments	Provide clear, understandable discharge instructions		
7. Collaboration with the health team			
Communicate the patient's pain and mobility concerns to the multidisciplinary team	Ensure all relevant information is shared with physiotherapists, doctors etc		
Coordinate with the physiotherapist for an appropriate rehabilitation plan	Ensure physiotherapy intervention is set up and tailored to the patient's needs		

8. Professionalism			
Maintain a calm, compassionate, and professional demeanor	Demonstrate confidence, professionalism and emotional intelligence		
Ensure privacy and dignity while assisting with care	Protect patient's dignity during assessments and interventions		
Follow hospital protocols for patient care and pain management	Adhere to established clinical guidelines and best practices		

⑩ 위급한 상태의 환자 관리

Station Ten: Managing the deteriorating patient

🖎 스테이션 목표

- Accurately assess the condition of a deteriorating patient and take appropriate immediate actions.
  악화된 환자의 상태를 정확히 평가하고, 적절한 즉각적인 조치를 취한다.

- Deliver clear and concise communication about the patient's condition to a doctor using the ISBAR framework. ISBAR(Identification, Situation, Background, Assessment, Recommendation)
  프레임워크를 사용하여 의사에게 명확하고 간결하게 환자의 상태를 전달한다.

- Maintain the patient's stability and prevent further deterioration.
  환자의 안정성을 유지하고 추가적인 악화를 방지한다.

- Understand and execute the doctor's instructions for follow-up care.
  의사의 지시를 이해하고, 필요한 후속 조치를 정확히 수행한다.

주요기술

1. Patient Assessment:

- Measure and interpret vital signs(respiratory rate, oxygen saturation, heart rate, blood pressure, etc.).
- Observe the patient's consciousness level, skin condition, and breathing pattern.
- Perform physical assessments, such as lung auscultation.

상태 평가 기술:

- 활력징후(호흡수, 산소포화도, 심박수, 혈압 등) 측정 및 해석.
- 환자의 의식 상태, 피부 상태, 호흡 패턴을 관찰.
- 폐 청진과 같은 신체 검진.

2. Immediate Nursing Interventions:

- Administer oxygen therapy(adjusting flow rate and checking the device).
- Adjust the patient's position(semi-Fowler's or high-Fowler's).
- Check IV lines and prepare for fluid administration if needed.

즉각적 간호 조치:

- 산소 요법 관리(유속 조정 및 장치 확인).
- 자세 조정(반좌위 또는 고좌위로 배치).
- IV 라인 점검 및 수액 치료 준비.

3. Communication Skills:

- Use the ISBAR framework to provide structured and clear information.
- Professionally explain the patient's condition and assessment findings.
- Confirm and clarify the doctor's instructions.

의사소통 능력:
- ISBAR 포맷을 활용한 명확하고 체계적인 정보 전달.
- 환자 상태와 평가 내용을 전문적으로 설명.
- 의사의 지시를 적극적으로 확인 및 실행.

4. Prioritization:

- Address life-threatening issues first.
- Perform all necessary nursing interventions before the doctor arrives.

우선순위 설정:
- 환자의 생명을 위협하는 요소를 우선적으로 관리.
- 의사의 개입 전, 가능한 모든 간호 조치 선행.

5. Documentation:

- Record changes in the patient's condition, interventions taken, and the doctor's instructions accurately.

문서화 기술:
- 환자의 상태 변화, 개입 조치, 의사의 지시를 정확히 기록.

평가기준

1. Patient Assessment:
- Were vital signs measured accurately, and abnormal values interpreted correctly?
- Were key symptoms and signs identified promptly?

환자 상태 평가:
- 활력징후를 정확히 측정하고, 비정상 수치를 올바르게 해석했는가?
- 환자의 주요 증상과 징후를 빠르게 확인했는가?

2. Interventions:
- Were appropriate nursing actions(oxygen therapy, positioning, etc.) taken immediately?
- Was prioritization of care appropriate to the patient's condition?

조치 및 개입:
- 적절한 간호 중재(산소 요법, 자세 조정 등)를 즉시 시행했는가?
- 상황에 맞는 우선순위를 설정했는가?

3. Communication:
- Was the ISBAR framework used systematically?
- Was the information delivered clearly, concisely, and confidently?

의사소통:
- ISBAR 프레임워크를 체계적으로 사용했는가?
- 명확하고 간결하며, 자신감 있게 의사에게 전달했는가?

4. Professionalism:
- Was the candidate calm, confident, and composed during the scenario?
- Was patient safety and well-being prioritized at all times?

전문성:
- 침착하고 자신감 있는 태도로 문제를 해결했는가?
- 환자 안전과 생명을 최우선으로 고려했는가?

5. Documentation:
- Were all interventions, observations, and communications recorded accurately?

문서화:
- 모든 조치와 관찰 내용을 정확히 기록했는가?

학습팁

1. Practice ISBAR Framework:
- Role-play using different scenarios to practice structured communication.
- Rehearse with colleagues to become comfortable presenting patient information clearly.

ISBAR 프레임워크 연습:
- 다양한 사례를 기반으로 ISBAR 구조에 맞춘 의사소통을 연습.
- 친구나 동료와 롤플레이를 통해 자연스럽게 전달하는 기술 습득.

2. Master Vital Signs Interpretation:

- Memorize normal ranges and identify abnormal values in various scenarios.
- For example, know what actions to take when oxygen saturation drops.

활력징후 해석 능력 강화:
- 정상 범위와 비정상 범위를 암기하고, 다양한 시나리오에서 변화의 의미를 이해.
  예를 들어, 산소포화도 저하가 나타날 때 즉각적인 조치를 떠올릴 수 있도록 연습

3. Simulate Emergency Situations:

- Practice quick decision-making under time constraints to manage a deteriorating patient.
- Focus on efficiently completing assessments, interventions, and communication within the time limit.

모의 상황에서 반응 속도 훈련:
- 제한된 시간 내에 상태 평가, 조치, 보고를 효과적으로 수행하는 연습.
- OSCE 시험에서 시간이 제한되므로 빠르고 정확한 판단 능력 필요

4. Understand Immediate Interventions:

- Familiarize yourself with oxygen therapy equipment (adjusting flow rates, nasal cannula, face mask usage).
- Practice patient positioning techniques to optimize respiratory function.

즉각적인 조치 이해:
- 산소 요법 장비 사용법(유속 조정, 비강 캐뉼라, 마스크 사용 등)을 숙지.
- 환자 자세 조정과 관련된 기본 간호기술 반복 연습.

5. Practice Auscultation:
↣ Use a stethoscope to differentiate lung sounds(e.g., crackles, wheezes) and understand their clinical significance.

청진 연습:
- 실제 청진기를 사용해 다양한 폐음(거품소리, 천명음 등)을 들어보고 차이를 구분하는 연습.
- 상태 변화의 근거를 빠르게 판단할 수 있도록 준비.

6. Effective Communication with Doctors:
↣ Reduce anxiety by practicing clear and concise delivery of critical points.
↣ Prepare notes with key points to stay organized during the handover.

7. 의사와의 의사소통:
- 의사소통 시 불안감을 줄이기 위해 명확하고 간결한 표현 연습.
- 중요 포인트를 간단히 메모하고, 전달 시 핵심 정보만 전달하는 연습

8. Develop Good Documentation Habits:

↳ Simulate documenting patient status changes, actions taken, and communication with the doctor.

문서화 습관 형성:
- 환자 상태 변화와 개입 내용을 체계적으로 기록하는 연습.
- ISBAR 후 전달한 내용과 환자의 반응을 문서화하는 시뮬레이션 진행.

9. Stay Updated on Guidelines:

↳ Review the latest ACLS (Advanced Cardiac Life Support), BLS (Basic Life Support) and guidelines for managing deteriorating patients.

가이드라인.숙지:
- 최신 ACLS(BLS 포함) 및 상태 악화 환자 관리 가이드라인을 참고해 최신 지식 유지.

ISBAR COMMUNICATION TOOL

I	Identify	➤ **Yourself:** 　☐ **name,** 　☐ **position,** 　☐ **location** ➤ **Receiver: Confirm who you are talking to** ➤ **Patient: name, age, sex, location**
S	Situation	➤ **State purpose "The reason I am calling is......."** ➤ **If urgent – SAY SO, Make it clear from the start** ➤ **May represent a summary of Assessment and Requirement**
B	Background	➤ **Tell the story** ➤ **Relevant information only:** 　☐ **history,** 　☐ **examination,** 　☐ **test results,** 　☐ **management** ➤ **If urgent: Relevant vital signs, current management**
A	Assessment	➤ **State what you think is going on, your interpretation** ➤ **Use ABCDE approach** 　☐ **Airway** 　☐ **Breathing** 　☐ **Circulation** 　☐ **Disability** 　☐ **Exposure** ➤ **State any interventions e.g applied oxygen**
R	Requirement	➤ **What you want from them – BE CLEAR** ➤ **State your request or requirement** 　☐ **Urgent review (state time frame)** 　☐ **Give approval / recommendation for further course of action while awaiting attendance eg. ECG, bloods** 　☐ **Give opinion on appropriate management**

Modified from Southern Health

✱ Exam Tips

- Stay Calm: Remain composed and focus on prioritizing patient safety to minimize errors.
- Time Management: Allocate time wisely; complete assessments and interventions within the 8-minute time frame.
- Patient Safety First: Ensure all actions are safe and appropriate for the patient's condition(e.g., checking oxygen equipment).
- Be Confident: Demonstrate confidence in both communication and nursing actions to reassure the examiner.

시험 팁:
- 침착함 유지: 긴장하지 말고 환자의 생명을 우선적으로 고려하며 실수를 줄이세요.
- 시간 관리: 각 단계에서 시간을 잘 분배하고, 8분 내에 환자 평가와 조치를 완료하세요.
- 환자 안전 중심: 환자의 안전을 고려해 모든 행동을 계획하세요(예: 산소 장비 확인).
- 자신감 있는 태도: 의사소통과 간호 시 자신감을 보여 평가자를 안심시킵니다.

✐ 예시

Background Information:

You are working as a registered nurse in a medical ward. The patient, Mr. John Smith(aged 65), was admitted two days ago with pneumonia. He has been receiving IV antibiotics and oxygen therapy via nasal prongs at 4L/min. Over the past hour, his condition appears to have deteriorated. His vital signs are abnormal, and his oxygen saturation has dropped. Your task is to assess the patient, escalate care to the doctor, and provide a clear handover using the ISBAR framework.

당신은 의료 병동에서 근무 중인 간호사입니다. 환자 존 스미스(65세)는 폐렴으로 이틀 전 입원했습니다. 그는 현재 IV 항생제와 4L/분의 산소 요법(비강 캐뉼라 사용)을 받고 있습니다. 최근 1시간 동안 상태가 악화된 것으로 보이며, 산소 포화도가 떨어졌습니다. 당신의 과제는 환자를 평가하고, 의사에게 환자의 상태를 보고하며, ISBAR 프레임워크를 사용해 명확하게 전달하는 것입니다.

Step 1: Patient Assessment

- **Visual Observation:** Patient appears pale, is breathing rapidly, and is drowsy.
- **Vital Signs:**
  - Respiratory rate: 30 breaths/min(normal: 12-20 breaths/min)
  - Heart rate: 120 bpm(tachycardic; normal: 60-100 bpm)
  - Blood pressure: 90/60 mmHg(hypotensive; normal: 120/80 mmHg)
  - Temperature: 38.5℃(febrile; normal: 36.1-37.2℃)
  - Oxygen saturation: 85% on 4L/min oxygen (normal: >94%)
- **Additional Findings:**
  - Chest auscultation reveals crackles in both lung bases.
  - Patient reports worsening shortness of breath and chest tightness.

1단계: 환자 평가
- **시각적 관찰:** 환자는 창백하고, 호흡이 빠르며, 졸린 상태입니다.
- **활력징후(Vital Signs):**
  · 호흡수: 30회/분(정상: 12-20회/분)
  · 심박수: 120회/분(빈맥; 정상: 60-100회/분)
  · 혈압: 90/60 mmHg(저혈압; 정상: 120/80 mmHg)
  · 체온: 38.5°C(발열; 정상: 36.1-37.2°C)
  · 산소 포화도(SpO2): 85%(4L/분 산소 요법; 정상: >94%)
- **추가 소견:**
  · 청진 시 양쪽 폐 기저부에서 거품소리가 들림.
  · 환자는 악화된 호흡곤란과 흉부 압박을 호소함.

Step 2: Intervention

1. Immediate Actions:

↪ Increase oxygen delivery to 6L/min via face mask and reassess SpO2.

↪ Position the patient in a high Fowler's position to ease breathing.

↪ Check IV line patency for potential fluid resuscitation.

↪ Attach continuous monitoring equipment(e.g., pulse oximetry, cardiac monitor).

↪ Initiate frequent observations(every 5 minutes).

1. 즉각적인 조치:
- 산소 공급을 6L/분으로 증가시키고 SpO2 재평가.
- 환자를 호흡이 편하도록 반좌위(High Fowler's position)로 자세 조정.
- 수액 치료를 위해 IV 라인 상태 점검.
- 맥박 산소계(pulse oximetry) 및 심박수 모니터링 장비 부착.
- 활력징후를 5분 간격으로 자주 관찰.

2. Prepare for Escalation:
- ↝ Collect and prepare relevant documents(e.g., patient chart, medication administration record).
- ↝ Gather necessary equipment in case of urgent intervention(e.g., suction, crash cart).

---

2. 보고 준비:
- 관련 문서(예: 환자 기록, 투약 기록)를 준비.
- 응급 처치에 필요한 장비(예: 석션 장치, 응급 카트) 준비.

Step 3: Handover to Doctor Using ISBAR

I - Identification:
"Hello, Dr. Taylor. My name is [Your Name], and I am the registered nurse caring for Mr. John Smith, a 65-year-old patient in Room 5."

I - Identification(신원 확인):
"안녕하세요, 테일러 의사님. 저는 [이름] 간호사입니다. 현재 존 스미스(65세) 환자를 간호하고 있으며, 이 환자는 병실 5번에 계십니다."

S - Situation:
"I am calling because Mr. Smith's condition is deteriorating. He was admitted with pneumonia but now has severe shortness of breath and low oxygen saturation despite increasing oxygen therapy."

S - Situation(상황):
"스미스 환자의 상태가 악화되어 연락드립니다. 폐렴으로 입원 중이었으나 현재 심한 호흡곤란과 산소포화도 저하를 보이고 있습니다."

B - Background:

"Mr. Smith was admitted two days ago for community-acquired pneumonia. He has been on IV antibiotics and oxygen at 4L/min via nasal prongs. He has no significant comorbidities, but he is now febrile at 38.5°C."

> **B - Background(배경):**
> "스미스 환자는 이틀 전 지역사회 획득 폐렴으로 입원하였고, IV 항생제와 4L/분의 산소 치료를 받고 있었습니다. 주요 동반질환은 없으며, 현재 체온이 38.5°C로 발열 상태입니다."

A - Assessment:

"His vital signs are concerning: respiratory rate of 30 breaths/min, heart rate of 120 bpm, blood pressure at 90/60 mmHg, temperature at 38.5°C, and oxygen saturation at 85% on 6L/min oxygen. Auscultation reveals crackles in both lung bases. I suspect he might be developing sepsis or worsening respiratory failure."

> **A - Assessment(평가):**
> "활력징후가 우려됩니다: 호흡수는 30회/분, 심박수는 120회/분, 혈압은 90/60 mmHg, 체온은 38.5°C, 산소포화도는 6L/분 산소 공급 시에도 85%입니다. 청진 시 양쪽 폐 기저부에서 거품소리가 들립니다. 패혈증(sepsis) 발생 또는 호흡부전이 악화된 것으로 의심됩니다."

R - Recommendation:

"I recommend that you assess Mr. Smith urgently. We may need to initiate higher-level oxygen support, consider fluid resuscitation, and order blood tests, including a full blood count, arterial blood gas analysis, and blood cultures. Do you have any other recommendations or instructions for now?"

R - Recommendation(권고):

"스미스 환자의 상태를 긴급히 평가해 주시길 권고드립니다. 더 높은 산소 요법, 수액 치료, 그리고 혈액 검사(예: CBC, 동맥혈 가스분석, 혈액 배양 검사)를 고려해야 할 것 같습니다. 현재 추가로 권고사항이 있으신가요?"

Step 4: Doctor's Response and Follow-Up

1. Listen and Document: Record the doctor's instructions clearly and act promptly on their orders.

2. Prepare for Further Actions:
- Ensure diagnostic tests are ordered and samples are collected(e.g., blood, sputum).
- Administer fluids or medications as prescribed.
- Notify the Rapid Response Team if the doctor instructs escalation to critical care.

3. Monitor Continuously: Keep observing the patient's condition and document any changes.

4단계: 의사의 응답 및 후속 조치
1. **듣고 기록하기**: 의사의 지시를 명확히 기록하고 신속히 실행.
2. **추가 조치 준비**:
   - 진단 검사가 주문된 경우 바로 실행(예: 혈액, 가래 채취).
   - 처방된 수액 또는 약물을 투여.
   - 의사의 지시에 따라 필요 시 신속대응팀(Rapid Response Team) 호출.
3. **지속적인 모니터링**: 환자의 상태 변화를 계속 관찰하고 문서화

Key Points to Demonstrate in the OSCE Station:
(OSCE 스테이션에서 보여줘야 할 핵심 사항)

- **Communication:** Clear and concise handover using the ISBAR format.
- **Prioritization:** Immediate actions to stabilize the patient(e.g., oxygen therapy, positioning).
- **Confidence and Professionalism:** Show a calm and composed demeanor when communicating with the doctor.
- **Documentation:** Accurately record the events, interventions, and doctor's instructions.

* **의사소통:** ISBAR 포맷을 사용하여 명확하고 간결하게 전달.
* **우선순위 설정:** 환자를 안정시키기 위한 즉각적인 조치(예: 산소 요법, 자세 조정).
* **자신감과 전문성:** 침착하고 전문적인 태도로 의사와 소통.
* **문서화:** 모든 사건, 개입 및 의사의 지시를 정확히 기록.

🡒 마킹 기준 체크리스트 Marking Criteria

Category	Step	Met	Not Met
1. initial assessment			
Perform hand hygiene and don gloves if required	Follow infection control protocols		
Introduce self and assess patient using ABCDE approach	Systematic evaluation of airway, breathing, circulation, disability and exposure		
Check vital signs and identify abnormalities	Measure BP, pulse, respiratory rate, oxygen saturation and temperature accurately		
Use appropriate monitoring equipment	Ensure correct usage of devices like pulse oximeter or ECG		
Recognise signs of clinical deterioration	Identify changes such as low oxygen levels, high pulse, or altered consciousness		
2. Immediate interventions			
Administer oxygen if required	Ensure proper oxygen delivery with the correct device and flow rate		
Position the patient appropriately	Maintain airway patency and ensure patient comfort		
Prepare emergency medication or fluids if prescribed	Follow safe medication administration protocols		
Escalate care promptly when necessary	Recognise the need for urgent intervention and contact the doctor		
3. Handover to Doctor			
Use ISBAR format for handover	Communicate situation, background, assessment, and recommendation		

Provide clear and concise information	Include key details such as patient identity, current issue and vital signs		
Report any interventions performed and patient response	Inform the doctor of steps already taken and their effectiveness		
Ask for and clarify any instructions given by the doctor	Ensure full understanding of next steps or further care		
4. Post-Handover Care			
Continue monitoring the patient	Regularly check vital signs and patient condition until the doctor arrives		
Document all actions and observations	Record interventions, patient responses, and details of the handover		
Ensure patient safety and comfort	Maintain proper positioning and administer any prescribed care		
5. Professionalism			
Maintain a calm and professional demeanor throughout	Demonstrate confidence and reassurance to the patient and team		
Communicate effectively with the patient	Explain actions to the patient and seek consent where possible		
Adhere to hospital protocols and guidelines	Ensure compliance with institutional safety and care standards		
Manage time efficiently	Complete the process promptly within the allocated time		

Part II

3장

10단계 예문과 단계별 1개 연습 시나리오

❶ 정신 건강 사정

Station 1: Mental Health Assessment

* Time: 10 minutes
* Setting: Post-operative care ward
* Patient: Mr. John Smith, 35 years old
* Presenting Complaint: depression and anxiety post operatively.

🖋 Example Scenario Description

Mr. John Smith, a 35-year-old male, was admitted following minor surgery. During routine postoperative care, Mr. Smith shared that he is experiencing feelings of depression and anxiety. He appears withdrawn and expresses difficulty sleeping since the procedure. As his nurse, you are tasked with conducting a mental health assessment to determine the severity of his symptoms, provide immediate emotional support, and develop a plan of care tailored to his needs.

> 존 스미스 씨(35세 남성)는 경미한 수술 후 입원했습니다. 수술 후 일반적인 간호 중, 스미스 씨는 우울감과 불안을 느낀다고 이야기했습니다. 그는 내성적인 모습을 보이며 수술 이후 수면에 어려움을 겪고 있다고 표현했습니다. 간호사로서, 당신은 그의 증상의 심각성을 평가하고 즉각적인 정서적 지원을 제공하며, 그의 필요에 맞춘 간호 계획을 수립해야 합니다.

Candidate Instructions:

1. Introduce Yourself and Explain the Assessment Process

- Approach Mr. Smith calmly and professionally, ensuring he feels comfortable and safe.
- Explain that you will ask some questions to better understand his emotional well-being and how you can support him during his recovery.
- Ensure that the conversation takes place in a private and quiet space to encourage openness and confidentiality.

> 스미스 씨에게 차분하고 전문적으로 접근하여 그가 편안하고 안전하다고 느낄 수 있도록 합니다. 그의 감정적 웰빙을 더 잘 이해하고 회복 과정에서 그를 어떻게 지원할 수 있는지 알기 위해 몇 가지 질문을 하겠다고 설명합니다. 대화가 개방적이고 개인정보 비밀이 유지될 수 있도록 조용하고 개인적인 공간에서 이루어지도록 합니다.

What to Say:
- "Hello, Mr. Smith, I'm [Your Name], one of the nurses looking after you today. I understand you've been feeling a bit down and anxious since your surgery. I'd like to ask you some questions about your emotional health so we can support you better. Is this a good time to talk?"

↳ "I want to assure you that everything you share will remain confidential within the care team. My goal is to help you feel more comfortable and supported."

- "안녕하세요, 스미스 씨. 저는 오늘 당신을 돌보는 간호사 [당신의 이름]입니다. 수술 후에 기분이 좀 가라앉고 불안감을 느끼고 계시다고 들었어요. 환자분의 감정 상태에 대해 몇 가지 질문을 드리고, 더 잘 지원해드리기 위해 노력하고 싶습니다. 지금 대화 나누기에 괜찮으신가요?"
- "환자분이 공유해주시는 모든 내용은 의료팀 내에서 비밀로 유지된다는 점을 안심시켜 드리고 싶습니다. 제 목표는 환자분이 더 편안하고 잘 지원받는다고 느끼실 수 있도록 돕는 것입니다."

2. Conduct a Comprehensive Mental Health assessment

2.1 Mood and Emotional State:

↳ Ask about his current mood and explore any feelings of sadness, anxiety, or hopelessness.

↳ Assess for signs of anhedonia(loss of interest in activities he usually enjoys).

- 현재 기분에 대해 물어보고 슬픔, 불안, 절망감 등의 감정을 살핍니다.
- 그가 보통 즐기던 활동에 흥미를 잃는 무쾌감(anhedonia) 징후가 있는지 평가합니다.

What to Say:

↳ "How have you been feeling emotionally since the surgery?"

↳ "Do you feel like you've lost interest in things you usually enjoy?"

> "수술 이후로 감정적으로 어떻게 느끼셨나요?", "평소에 즐기던 것들에 흥미를 잃었다고 느끼시나요?"

2.2 Thought Processes and Perception:

- Inquire about any negative thoughts, feelings of guilt, or worthlessness.
- Ask if he has experienced any intrusive thoughts or unusual perceptions

> - 부정적인 생각, 죄책감, 무가치감을 느낀 적이 있는지 질문합니다.
> - 침투적 사고나 비정상적인 인식을 경험했는지 물어봅니다.

What to Say:

- "Have you been having any negative or distressing thoughts?"
- "Do you ever feel overwhelmed by feelings of guilt or worry?"

> - "부정적이거나 괴로운 생각을 해본 적이 있나요?"
> - "죄책감이나 걱정으로 압도당한 적이 있나요?"

2.3 Behaviour and Daily Functioning:

- Discuss how his emotional state is affecting his appetite, sleep, and energy levels.
- Ask about his ability to perform everyday tasks or maintain relationships.

> - 그의 감정 상태가 식욕, 수면, 에너지 수준에 어떤 영향을 미치는지 논의하세요.
> - 일상적인 작업을 수행하거나 인간관계를 유지하는 능력에 대해 물어보세요.

What to Say:

⇝ "Have you noticed any changes in your appetite or sleep since the surgery?"

⇝ "Do you feel like your energy levels have been lower than usual?"

> "수술 이후 식욕이나 수면에 변화가 있었나요?", "에너지 수준이 평소보다 낮아진 것처럼 느껴지시나요?"

3. Risk Factors and Safety Assessment:

⇝ Evaluate if he has experienced any thoughts of self-harm or suicide.

⇝ Ask if he has a support system, such as family or friends,, and determine their involvement in his recovery.

> - 그가 자해나 자살에 대한 생각을 한 적이 있는지 평가합니다.
> - 가족이나 친구와 같은 지지 체계가 있는지 물어보고, 그들이 그의 회복에 얼마나 관여하고 있는지 확인합니다.

What to Say:

⇝ "Sometimes when people feel down, they may have thoughts of hurting themselves. Have you experienced any thoughts like that?"

⇝ "Do you have friends or family members you can rely on for support?"

> "가끔 사람들이 우울할 때 자신을 해치고 싶은 생각을 할 수도 있습니다. 그런 생각을 해본 적이 있으신가요?", "기댈 수 있는 친구나 가족이 있으신가요?"

4. Provide Emotional Support and Immediate Interventions

- Reassure him that his feelings are valid and that support is available.
- Offer relaxation techniques, such as deep breathing exercises, to help manage his anxiety.
- Suggest resources for further support, such as the hospital's mental health team or counselling services.

> 그의 감정이 정상적이며 지원이 가능하다는 점을 안심시켜 주세요.
> 심호흡 운동과 같은 이완 기법을 제공하여 불안을 관리하도록 도와주세요.
> 병원의 정신 건강팀이나 상담 서비스와 같은 추가 지원을 위한 자원을 제안하세요.

What to Say:

- "Thank you for sharing how you've been feeling. I want you to know that what you're going through is completely valid, and we're here to support you."
- "Would you like me to arrange a visit with our mental health specialist or a counsellor to talk further about what you're experiencing?"

> - "환자분의 감정을 함께 공유해 주셔서 감사합니다. 환자분이 겪고 있는 일이 완전히 정상적인 일임을 알려드리고 싶으며, 저희는 당신을 지원하기 위해 여기 있습니다."
> - "정신건강 전문가나 상담사와 만나서 현재 겪고 있는 일에 대해 더 이야기해보는 자리를 마련해 드릴까요?"

5. Notify the Healthcare Team and Develop a Plan of Care

- Document the findings of your assessment, including his reported symptoms, mood, and any identified risk factors.
- Notify the physician and mental health team for further evaluation if needed.
- Develop a plan of care that includes emotional support, monitoring, and referrals to appropriate services.

> 평가 결과를 문서화하여 환자가 보고한 증상, 기분, 그리고 확인된 위험 요인을 포함하십시오. 필요한 경우 추가 평가를 위해 의사와 정신건강 팀에 알리십시오. 정서적 지원, 모니터링, 그리고 적절한 서비스로의 의뢰를 포함하는 간호 계획을 수립하십시오.

What to Document:

"Mr. Smith reports feeling depressed and anxious since surgery, with difficulty sleeping and low energy levels. He denies thoughts of self-harm but expresses feelings of hopelessness. Will refer to the mental health team for further evaluation and provide ongoing emotional support."

Key Points to Remember:

- Ensure Mr. Smith feels heard and supported during the assessment.
- Assess mood, behavior, thought processes, and safety in a structured manner.
- Provide reassurance and practical resources for managing his emotional health.
- Collaborate with the healthcare team to ensure Mr. Smith receives comprehensive care.

Example Interaction:

Nurse: "Good morning, Mr. Smith. My name is [Nurse's Name], and I am one of the nurses here. I understand you've been feeling a bit down and anxious lately. Is it okay if we talk about how you've been feeling? This will help us understand what support you might need."

Mr. Smith: "Yes, that's fine. I've just been feeling really low and anxious since my surgery."

Nurse: "I'm sorry to hear that. Can you tell me more about your mood? How have you been feeling most of the time?"

Mr. Smith: "I've been feeling very down, like there's no point in anything. It's been going on for a few weeks now."

Nurse: "I understand. Have you noticed any changes in your sleep patterns or appetite recently?"

Mr. Smith: "Yes, I've had trouble sleeping, and I haven't been eating much."

Nurse: "Have you experienced any feelings of hopelessness or thoughts of harming yourself?"

Mr. Smith: "Sometimes I feel like I don't want to be here anymore, but I haven't made any plans."

Nurse: "Thank you for sharing that with me. It's really important that we address these feelings. I'm here to help, and we'll make sure you get the support you need."

Nurse: "Do you have any support from family or friends at the moment?"

Mr. Smith: "I do, but I haven't really talked to them about how I'm feeling."

Nurse: "It's good to know you have support available. We'll work together to help you feel better. I'll make a note of our conversation and suggest some steps we can take from here, including speaking with our mental health team."

✍ Documentation example

Date and Time

Patient states, "I feel down most of the time lately." Reports difficulty concentrating and a lack of interest in activities they used to enjoy. Denies hallucinations, delusions, or suicidal ideation. The patient describes issues with sleep and reduced appetite.

Patient appears well-groomed and is cooperative during the assessment. Eye contact was maintained throughout. Speech is clear and coherent with a normal rate and tone. Affect appears restricted but appropriate to the situation. No signs of agitation or psychomotor slowing were observed.

Patient presents with mild depressive symptoms, as evidenced by low mood, reduced interest, and difficulty concentrating. No immediate safety concerns were identified during the assessment.

Plan:

1. Provide reassurance and discuss available support options.
2. Refer to GP for evaluation and possible intervention for sleep and appetite concerns.
3. Follow-up in 2 weeks to monitor progress.
4. Encourage patient to use self-care strategies, such as relaxation techniques and engaging in physical activity.

Signature: Your name and designation

연습 Scenario 1:
Excessive anxiety and worry

* Time: 10 minutes
* Setting: Outpatient Clinic
* Patient: Ms. Jane Doe, 28 years old
* Presenting Complaint: Excessive anxiety and worry

Example Scenario Description:

Ms. Jane Doe, a 28-year-old female, presents to the outpatient clinic for a follow-up appointment. She reports that for the past six months, she has been experiencing persistent anxiety and excessive worry about various aspects of her life, including work, relationships, and personal health. These symptoms are affecting her daily functioning, and she has difficulty relaxing. Ms. Doe expresses concerns about her mental health and feels overwhelmed by her constant state of worry. As a nurse, you are tasked with conducting a comprehensive mental health assessment to understand the severity of her symptoms and formulate an appropriate care plan to provide support.

Candidate Instructions:

1. Introduce Yourself and Explain the Purpose of the Assessment

- Greet the patient warmly and introduce yourself to build rapport.
- Explain the purpose of the mental health assessment, emphasizing the importance of understanding her anxiety symptoms and creating a supportive care plan.

What to say:
- "Hi Ms. Doe, my name is [Your Name], and I'll be conducting a mental health assessment today to better understand what you've been experiencing with your anxiety. This will help us work together on a plan to support your well-being."
- "It's important for me to understand how your anxiety is affecting you, so please feel free to share openly. This will help guide us in finding the right solutions."

2. Conduct a Thorough Mental Health Assessment

- Ask open-ended questions to explore the patient's anxiety symptoms, their triggers, and impact on her daily life.

- Assess the duration, frequency, and intensity of her symptoms(e.g., restlessness, difficulty concentrating, irritability, sleep disturbances).
- Explore her coping mechanisms and any current treatments or strategies she may be using to manage her anxiety(e.g., therapy, medications, relaxation techniques).
- Screen for any signs of depression, panic attacks, or other comorbid mental health conditions that may require attention.

What to say:
- "Can you tell me a bit more about how your anxiety has been affecting you recently? Are there any specific situations that tend to trigger your anxiety?"
- "How often do you feel this way? Are there any physical symptoms, like restlessness, muscle tension, or trouble sleeping, that you've noticed?"
- "How are you coping with these feelings, and are there any strategies or support you've been using so far?"
- "Do you also experience any other emotions, such as sadness or loss of interest, that we should be aware of?"

3. Document Findings and Determine a Plan of Care
- Record all relevant details from the assessment, including the severity and frequency of anxiety

symptoms, any signs of depression or other concerns, and the patient's coping strategies.
- Identify immediate interventions that could help reduce symptoms, such as relaxation techniques, mindfulness exercises, or referral to a mental health professional.
- Suggest follow-up appointments and potential resources for mental health support, such as therapy or counselling services.

What to say(for documentation):
- "I'll document everything we've discussed today so that we have a comprehensive record of your symptoms and the steps we'll take moving forward. This will include any support resources we recommend, as well as next steps in your care."

4. Educate the Patient and Provide Support
- Offer practical strategies for managing anxiety, including deep breathing exercises, mindfulness, and stress management techniques.
- Encourage Ms. Doe to practice self-care and to reach out for support if her symptoms worsen.
- Provide her with educational resources or referrals to mental health professionals as needed.
- Assure her that seeking help is a positive step towards improving her mental well-being.

What to say:

- "I'd like to share a few strategies that might help you manage your anxiety. For instance, deep breathing and mindfulness exercises can be really calming in stressful moments. Would you like me to guide you through one of these now?"
- "It's also important to reach out for support when you need it, and we can help connect you with a therapist or counsellor if that's something you're open to."
- "Remember, anxiety is something we can work together on, and taking these small steps is a positive way to start feeling more in control."

❷ 신체사정(활력징후 측정)

Station two: Physiological assessment

* Time: 10 minutes
* Setting: General practice clinic
* Patient: Mr. John Smith, 55 years old
* Presenting Complaint: Shortness of breath and persistent cough

✐ Example Scenario Description:

You are a registered nurse in a general practice clinic. Mr. John Smith, a 55-year-old male, has presented with complaints of shortness of breath and a persistent cough that has lasted for several weeks. He reports that his symptoms have gradually worsened, and he occasionally experiences chest tightness, especially at night. He has no known history of asthma but has been a smoker for 30 years. He denies any recent fever or upper respiratory infections but mentions that his sputum has been slightly discoloured.

Your task is to conduct a comprehensive respiratory assessment, identify any potential concerns, and determine the appropriate next steps for his care. You will need to evaluate his symptoms, perform a focused physical examination, and discuss a possible plan of care.

> 당신은 일반 진료 클리닉에서 근무하는 간호사입니다. 55세 남성인 John Smith 씨가 숨이 가쁘고 몇 주째 지속되는 기침 증상으로 내원했습니다. 그는 증상이 점차 악화되었으며, 특히 밤에 가슴이 조이는 느낌이 가끔 있다고 보고했습니다. 그는 천식 병력이 없지만, 30년 동안 흡연을 해왔습니다. 그는 최근에 열이나 상기도 감염 증상이 없었다고 부인하지만, 가래 색이 약간 변했다고 언급했습니다.
> Candidate의 임무는 포괄적인 호흡기 평가를 수행하여 잠재적인 문제를 파악하고 적절한 다음 단계를 결정하는 것입니다. 환자의 증상을 평가하고, 집중적인 신체 검사를 실시하며, 가능한 간호 계획을 논의해야 합니다.

◈ Candidate Instructions:

1. Introduce Yourself and Establish Rapport

- Greet Mr. Smith warmly and introduce yourself.
- Explain the purpose of the assessment and ensure he is comfortable discussing his symptoms.
- Obtain consent before proceeding with the examination.

> Smith 씨에게 따뜻하게 인사하고 자신을 소개합니다. 평가의 목적을 설명하고, 증상에 대해 편안하게 이야기할 수 있도록 합니다. 검사를 진행하기 전에 동의를 받습니다

What to say:

"Hello, Mr. Smith, my name is [Your Name], and I am one of the nurses here today. I understand you have been experiencing shortness of breath and a persistent cough. I'd like to ask you some questions and conduct a respiratory assessment to better understand your condition. Does that sound okay to you?"

"Everything we discuss will remain confidential within the care team. My goal is to ensure we provide you with the best possible care."

> "안녕하세요, Smith 씨. 저는 오늘 여기에서 근무하는 간호사 [본인 이름]입니다.
> 숨이 가쁘고 지속적인 기침 증상이 있다고 들었습니다. 상태를 더 잘 이해하기 위해 몇 가지 질문을 드리고 호흡기 평가를 진행하고자 하는데 괜찮으신가요?"
> "우리가 나누는 모든 이야기는 의료 팀 내에서만 비밀로 유지됩니다. 저의 목표는 최상의 치료를 제공해 드리는 것입니다."

2. Conduct a Thorough Respiratory Assessment

2.1 History Taking

- Ask about the onset, duration, and progression of his symptoms.
- Determine any aggravating or relieving factors.
- Inquire about his smoking history and exposure to environmental irritants.
- Ask about past medical history, including any respiratory conditions or chronic diseases.
- Check for associated symptoms such as fever, wheezing, fatigue, or weight loss.

> - 증상의 시작 시기, 지속 기간 및 진행 상태에 대해 질문합니다.
> - 증상을 악화시키거나 완화하는 요인을 확인합니다.
> - 흡연력 및 환경적 자극물 노출 여부를 조사합니다.
> - 호흡기 질환이나 만성 질환 등 과거 병력을 확인합니다.
> - 발열, 천명(쌕쌕거림), 피로, 체중 감소 등의 관련 증상이 있는지 확인합니다.

What to say:

"Can you describe when your symptoms started and how they have changed over time?"

"Have you noticed anything that makes your breathing worse or better?"

"Do you have any history of respiratory conditions, such as asthma or chronic bronchitis?"

"Have you had any recent infections, fever, or night sweats?"

> "증상이 언제 시작되었고 시간이 지나면서 어떻게 변했는지 설명해 주시겠어요?"
> "호흡을 더 나빠지게 하거나 좋아지게 하는 요인이 있나요?"
> "천식이나 만성 기관지염 같은 호흡기 질환 병력이 있으신가요?"
> "최근에 감염이나 발열, 야간 발한을 경험한 적이 있으신가요?"

2.1 Physical Examination

- Measure and record vital signs, including respiratory rate, oxygen saturation, heart rate, and blood pressure.
- Observe for signs of respiratory distress, such as accessory muscle use, nasal flaring, or cyanosis.
- Perform auscultation of the lungs to assess for wheezing, crackles, or diminished breath sounds.
- Assess chest expansion and symmetry.
- Check for peripheral signs such as clubbing or cyanosis.

- 호흡수, 산소포화도, 심박수, 혈압 등 생명징후를 측정하고 기록합니다.
- 보조호흡 근육 사용, 코벌링임 증상, 청색증 등의 호흡곤란 징후를 관찰합니다.
- 폐의 청진을 통해 천명음, 기침소리, 또는 숨소리 감소 등을 사정합니다.
- 가슴 팽창 및 대칭을 평가합니다.
- 손톱끝 변형이나 청색증을 확인하여 말초혈관 상태를 봅니다.

What to say:
- "I'm going to check your vital signs and listen to your lungs to assess how well you're breathing."
- "Take a deep breath in and out for me, please. Let me know if you feel any discomfort."

"저는 이제 생명징후를 확인하고, 호흡이 잘 되고 있는지 평가하기 위해 폐소리를 들을 거예요.", "깊게 숨을 들이쉬고 내쉬어 주세요. 불편한 느낌이 있으면 말씀해 주세요."

3. Document Findings and Develop a Plan of Care

- Record all assessment findings, including reported symptoms, physical examination results, and any risk factors identified.
- Notify the physician if there are signs of respiratory compromise or potential underlying conditions such as COPD or pneumonia.
- Provide initial management recommendations, such as smoking cessation support, breathing exercises, or inhaler use if appropriate
- Arrange for further diagnostic tests, such as a chest X-ray, pulmonary function tests, or sputum analysis if indicated.

- 보고된 증상, 신체검사 결과, 식별된 위험 요소 등을 포함한 모든 평가 결과를 기록합니다.
- 호흡 기능 저하나 COPD, 폐렴과 같은 잠재적인 기저 질환의 징후가 있을 경우 의사에게 알립니다.
- 적절하다면 흡연 중단 지원, 호흡 운동, 흡입기 사용 등의 초기 관리 권장 사항을 제공합니다.
- 필요한 경우 흉부 엑스레이, 폐 기능 검사, 객담 분석과 같은 추가 진단 검사를 준비합니다.

What to say:

↪ "Based on my assessment, I will document my findings and discuss them with the physician. They may recommend further tests or treatments."

↪ "Since you mentioned a history of smoking and persistent symptoms, we may consider additional tests to check your lung function."

↪ "Would you like some information on smoking cessation programs and breathing exercises that might help improve your symptoms?"

"제가 진행한 사정을 바탕으로 찾아낸 사항을 문서화하고 의사와 논의할 예정입니다. 의사분들이 추가 검사나 치료를 권할 수 있습니다.", "흡연 경력과 지속적인 증상을 언급하셨기 때문에, 폐 기능을 확인하기 위한 추가 검사를 고려할 수 있습니다.", "흡연 중단 프로그램이나 증상 개선에 도움이 될 수 있는 호흡 운동에 대한 정보를 원하시면 알려드릴 수 있습니다."

Documentation example

Date/Time

Patient presented with complaints of shortness of breath(SOB) and a persistent cough lasting approximately two weeks. He reports the cough is dry and worse at night. Denies chest pain, fever, or recent illnesses. States SOB is more noticeable during physical activity, such as walking up stairs. No history of asthma or known lung conditions. Smokes approximately 10 cigarettes per day for the last 30 years.

Vital Signs; for example,
- Temperature: 36.8°C
- Pulse: 92 bpm, regular
- Respiratory Rate: 22 breaths/min
- Blood Pressure: 138/86 mmHg
- SpO2: 94% on room air

Physical Examination; for example,
- Inspection: Mild dyspnea noted; no cyanosis or accessory muscle use.
- Palpation: Equal chest expansion bilaterally; no tenderness.
- Percussion: Resonant sounds bilaterally.
- Auscultation: Bilateral lung fields clear; no wheezes, crackles, or rhonchi.

Assessment; for example,
- Persistent dry cough and mild dyspnoea on exertion.
- Oxygen saturation slightly decreased.
- Potential contributing factors: smoking history and possible environmental irritants.

Plan:
1. Educate patients on smoking cessation resources and the impact of smoking on respiratory health.
2. Recommend chest X-ray to rule out underlying conditions(e.g., chronic obstructive pulmonary disease, interstitial lung disease).
3. Provide a prescription for a short-term bronchodilator if symptoms persist.
4. Suggest saline nasal spray or humidifier for nighttime symptom relief.
5. Advise follow-up appointment in one week to reassess symptoms and discuss test results.
6. Encourage increased fluid intake and rest.

Signature: name, RN

연습 Scenario 1:
Chest pain

* Time: 10 minutes
* Setting: Emergency Department
* Patient: Ms. Emily Brown, 60 years old
* Presenting Complaint: Chest pain

Example Scenario Description:

Ms. Emily Brown, a 60-year-old female, has presented to the emergency department complaining of chest pain. She reports that the pain began two hours ago while she was walking and has been intermittent, with a sensation of pressure in the centre of her chest. She also mentions feeling slightly short of breath and nauseous. Your task is to conduct a thorough cardiovascular assessment to identify any potential underlying causes, such as acute coronary syndrome(ACS), and provide appropriate care based on your findings.

Candidate Instructions:

1. Introduce Yourself and Explain the Purpose of the Assessment

- Greet Ms. Brown calmly and reassuringly to establish rapport.
- Explain the purpose of the cardiovascular assessment and inform her that you will be asking questions and performing a physical exam to help identify the cause of her chest pain.

What to say:
- "Hello Ms. Brown, my name is [Your Name], and I'm a nurse here in the emergency department. I understand you're experiencing chest pain, and I'm going to ask you some questions and perform an assessment to determine what might be causing it."
- "This will help us provide the best care possible for you. Is it alright if I ask you some questions about your symptoms?"

2. Perform a Thorough Cardiovascular Assessment
History Taking:
- Ask Ms. Brown to describe the onset, duration, and intensity of the chest pain(e.g., sharp, dull, pressure-like).
- Inquire about any radiation of the pain(e.g., to the arm, jaw, back).

- Ask about any associated symptoms, such as nausea, sweating, dizziness, or shortness of breath.
- Take her medical history, including any past cardiac events, risk factors(e.g., hypertension, diabetes, smoking, family history of heart disease), and current medications.

Physical Examination:
- Assess vital signs(blood pressure, heart rate, respiratory rate, oxygen saturation).
- Listen for heart murmurs or irregularities and assess for signs of heart failure(e.g., peripheral oedema, jugular venous distension).
- Perform a focused cardiovascular examination, including palpation of pulses and auscultation for any abnormal heart sounds.

Key Questions to Ask:
- "Can you describe the pain? Is it sharp, dull, or a feeling of pressure?"
- "Does the pain radiate anywhere, like to your arm, jaw, or back?"
- "Have you noticed any other symptoms, such as nausea, sweating, or shortness of breath?"
- "Do you have any history of heart disease, hypertension, or diabetes?"
- "Are you currently taking any medications for heart-related conditions?"

3. Document Findings and Develop a Plan of Care

- Document Ms. Brown's reported symptoms, including the onset, quality, and location of the chest pain, as well as any associated symptoms.
- Record her vital signs, including blood pressure, heart rate, respiratory rate, and oxygen saturation.
- Include findings from the physical examination, such as any abnormal heart sounds, and the results of your history taking.
- Based on your assessment, suggest further diagnostic tests, such as an ECG, chest X-ray, or cardiac biomarkers, and prepare for possible interventions(e.g., nitro-glycerine administration, oxygen therapy, or preparing for transfer to a cardiology team).
- Prepare for the possible escalation of care if ACS or another serious cardiovascular condition is suspected.

What to say(for documentation):

- "Patient reports chest pain described as pressure-like, starting two hours ago, with associated shortness of breath and nausea. Vital signs: BP 150/90 mmHg, HR 98 bpm, RR 18, SpO2 95%. ECG ordered for further assessment."
- "Cardiac history: Patient has a history of hypertension, no prior heart attack. No known allergies. Preparing for possible medication administration and further diagnostic workup."

4. Communicate Findings and Plan of Care

↳ After documenting your findings, communicate the situation with the physician and other relevant team members, ensuring that the necessary tests and interventions are initiated promptly.

↳ Update Ms. Brown on the steps being taken, explaining that you will need to perform further tests to determine the cause of her symptoms.

What to say to the patient:

↳ "Ms. Brown, I'm going to share this information with the doctor, and we'll do some additional tests, like an ECG, to help us better understand what's going on. I will keep you informed throughout the process, and we're here to make sure you get the care you need."

↳ "If the pain gets worse or you start feeling shorter of breath, please let me know immediately."

5. Complete Documentation and Follow-Up Plan

↳ Ensure that the assessment, findings, and the plan of care are thoroughly documented in the patient's record.

↳ Include any interventions provided, such as administering oxygen or nitroglycerin if prescribed, and note the plan for further diagnostic workup or referrals.

↳ Clearly document the follow-up plan, including when the physician will be consulted and when further diagnostics will be performed.

What to say(for documentation):
↳ "Patient to undergo ECG and labs to rule out myocardial infarction. Ongoing monitoring of vitals. Cardiology to be consulted for further management."

❸ 세부 생리학적 사정

Specific physiological assessment

* Time: 10 minutes
* Setting: Orthopaedic Surgical Ward
* Situation: Recognizing and assessing symptoms of Deep Vein Thrombosis(DVT) and Pulmonary Embolism (PE)

✐ Example Scenario Description:

You are a registered nurse working in an Orthopaedic Surgical ward. Your patient, Mrs. Sarah Thompson, a 65-year-old female, has recently undergone total knee replacement surgery and has been immobile for a few days. She is now experiencing pain and swelling in one of her legs, along with shortness of breath. You suspect she may be experiencing symptoms of DVT and/or PE, and you must assess the patient appropriately.

Your task is to effectively assess the patient's symptoms, perform the necessary physiological assessments to detect DVT or PE, and communicate with the medical team about the findings.

당신은 정형외과 외과 병동에서 근무하는 간호사입니다. 당신의 환자인 사라 톰슨(Sarah Thompson) 씨는 65세 여성으로, 최근 무릎 전치환술(total knee replacement) 수술을 받았으며, 며칠 동안 움직이지 못했습니다. 현재 그녀는 한쪽 다리에 통증과 부종을 호소하며, 숨이 가쁜 증상을 보이고 있습니다. 당신은 그녀가 심부정맥혈전증(DVT) 및/또는 폐색전증(PE)의 증상을 보이고 있다고 의심하며, 환자의 상태를 적절하게 평가해야 합니다.

간호사로써 당신의 임무는 환자의 증상을 효과적으로 평가하고, DVT 또는 PE를 감지하기 위한 필요한 생리학적 평가를 수행하며, 의료진에게 소견을 전달하는 것입니다.

Candidate Instructions:

Step 1: Patient Communication and Preparation

1.1 Introduce Yourself and Confirm Identity

↳ Knock on the door, greet the patient, and check their identity.

What to say:

↳ "Good morning, Mrs. Thompson. My name is [Your Name], and I am your nurse today. Could you please confirm your full name and date of birth? Thank you."

좋은 아침입니다, 톰슨 씨. 저는 오늘 담당 간호사 [본인의 이름]입니다. 성함과 생년월일을 확인해 주시겠어요? 감사합니다."

1.2 Explain the Procedure and Obtain Consent

↳ Explain the importance of assessing for symptoms of DVT and PE, as well as the physical examination you will perform.

What to say:

↳ "I need to check your legs for signs of a condition called deep vein thrombosis, which can cause swelling, pain, and redness. I'll also assess your breathing and listen to your chest to rule out pulmonary embolism. You may feel a bit of pressure during the exam, but it shouldn't be painful. Do you have any questions or concerns before we begin?"

> "다리에서 부종, 통증, 발적을 유발할 수 있는 심부정맥혈전증(DVT) 징후가 있는지 확인해야 합니다. 또한 폐색전증(PE)을 배제하기 위해 호흡 상태를 평가하고 가슴 소리를 청진할 것입니다. 검사 중 약간의 압력을 느낄 수 있지만 통증이 있지는 않을 것입니다. 시작하기 전에 궁금한 점이나 걱정되는 사항이 있으신가요?"

: Obtain verbal consent before proceeding.

1.3 Ensure Patient Comfort and Positioning
↪ Ask the patient to lie down or sit comfortably, ensuring their legs are accessible for examination.

What to say:
↪ "Please lie back in bed so I can examine your legs and listen to your chest."

Step 2: Equipment Preparation and Aseptic Technique
2.1 Perform Hand Hygiene and Wear PPE
↪ Wash hands thoroughly and wear gloves if necessary. Ensure aseptic technique if touching any areas of potential infection or injury.

> 손을 깨끗이 씻고 필요하면 장갑을 착용합니다. 감염이나 부상의 위험이 있는 부위를 만질 경우 무균 기술을 유지해야 합니다.

What to say:
➢ "I'm now washing my hands and putting on gloves to ensure cleanliness during the exam."

Step 3: Assessment of Deep Vein Thrombosis (DVT)

3.1 Inspect the Leg for Signs of DVT
➢ Inspect the affected leg for signs of redness, swelling, or any visible distended veins. DVT usually occurs in the lower extremities.

> **심부정맥혈전증(DVT) 징후에 대한 다리 검사**
> 영향을 받은 다리를 검사하여 발적, 부기 또는 확장된 정맥이 보이는지 확인합니다. DVT는 일반적으로 하체에서 발생합니다.

What to say:
➢ "I'm going to inspect your legs to check for any signs of redness, swelling, or visible veins."

> "다리에 발적, 부기 또는 확장된 정맥이 있는지 확인하기 위해 검사를 진행하겠습니다."

3.2 Palpate the Leg for Tenderness
➢ Gently palpate along the calf, thigh, and ankle for any areas of tenderness, warmth, or swelling. Be sure to use your fingers to avoid unnecessary pressure.

> 종아리, 허벅지, 발목을 따라 부드럽게 촉진하여 압통, 따뜻한 감각 또는 부기가 있는지 확인합니다. 불필요한 압력을 피하기 위해 손가락을 사용하여 검사합니다.

What to say:

↬ "I will gently palpate your leg to see if you feel any tenderness or warmth, which can be a sign of clotting."

> "다리에 부드럽게 촉진하여 압통이나 따뜻한 감각이 있는지 확인하겠습니다. 이는 혈전의 징후일 수 있습니다."

3.3 Perform the Homan's Sign Test

↬ Flex the patient's foot upward towards the shin while the leg is extended. This maneuver may provoke pain if DVT is present, although this test is not always reliable.

> **호만 징후 검사를 수행합니다.**
> 환자의 다리를 편 상태에서 발을 정강이 쪽으로 위로 굽힙니다. 이 동작이 통증을 유발하면 DVT가 있을 가능성이 있지만, 이 검사는 항상 신뢰할 수 있는 것은 아닙니다.

What to say:

↬ "I'm going to gently flex your foot upward to check for any pain, which could be a sign of deep vein thrombosis."

> "제가 발을 부드럽게 위로 굽혀서 통증이 있는지 확인하겠습니다. 통증이 느껴진다면 심부정맥혈전증의 징후일 수 있습니다."

Step 4: Assessment for Pulmonary Embolism (PE)

4.1 Assess for Shortness of Breath (SOB)
➢ Ask the patient if they are experiencing any shortness of breath, especially when resting or during mild exertion.

환자에게 휴식 중이거나 가벼운 활동 중에 숨이 차는 느낌이 있는지 물어보세요.

What to say:
➢ "Are you feeling short of breath, especially when you're lying down or after minimal activity?"

"누워 있을 때나 가벼운 활동 후에 숨이 차는 느낌이 드시나요?"

4.2 Inspect the Chest for Tachypnoea
➢ Observe the patient's breathing rate for signs of tachypnoea (rapid breathing), which may indicate difficulty breathing due to PE.

환자의 호흡 속도를 관찰하여 빈호흡(빠른 호흡) 징후가 있는지 확인합니다. 이는 폐색전증(PE)으로 인한 호흡 곤란을 나타낼 수 있습니다.

What to say:
➢ "I'm checking your breathing rate to see if it's faster than normal, which can sometimes happen with pulmonary embolism."

"폐색전증이 있을 때 호흡이 평소보다 빨라질 수 있기 때문에 지금 호흡 속도를 확인하겠습니다."

4.3 Measure Oxygen Saturation
↳ Use a pulse oximeter to measure oxygen saturation. A low oxygen saturation level may indicate PE.

> 펄스 옥시미터를 사용하여 산소 포화도를 측정하겠습니다. 낮은 산소 포화도는 폐색전증을 나타낼 수 있습니다.

What to say:
↳ "I'm going to check your oxygen levels now to ensure you're breathing adequately."

> "이제 산소 수치를 확인하여 충분히 호흡하고 계신지 확인하겠습니다."

4.4 Auscultate the Lungs
↳ Listen to the patient's lungs for abnormal breath sounds, such as crackles or wheezing, which may indicate a PE. A clear lung sound does not rule out PE, but it is important to rule out other potential causes.

> 환자의 폐에서 이상 호흡음(수포음 또는 천명음 등)이 있는지 확인합니다. 폐색전증이 있더라도 폐음이 정상일 수 있지만, 다른 가능한 원인을 배제하는 것이 중요합니다.

What to say:
↳ "I'm going to listen to your lungs to make sure there are no abnormal sounds that might suggest a pulmonary issue."

> "폐에 이상 소리가 있는지 확인하기 위해 청진하겠습니다."

Step 5: Post-Assessment Care and Patient Education

5.1 Dispose of Used Equipment Properly
- Dispose of any gloves, tissues, or swabs used during the assessment into the appropriate waste container.

사용한 장갑, 휴지 또는 면봉을 적절한 폐기물 용기에 버리십시오.

What to say:
- "I'm disposing of any used materials now to maintain cleanliness."

"지금 사용한 물품들을 처분하여 청결을 유지하겠습니다."

5.2 Monitor for Changes or Complications
- Encourage the patient to notify you if they experience sudden chest pain, worsening shortness of breath, or calf pain.

환자에게 갑작스러운 흉통, 악화되는 호흡곤란 또는 종아리 통증이 발생하면 즉시 알리도록 권장하세요.

What to say:
- "Please let me know immediately if you experience sudden chest pain, increased shortness of breath, or if the pain in your leg gets worse."

"갑작스러운 흉통, 호흡곤란이 심해지거나 다리 통증이 악화되면 즉시 알려주세요."

5.3 Provide Patient Education on Symptoms to Monitor
↪ Educate the patient on the importance of monitoring for signs of complications, including chest pain, difficulty breathing, or swelling in the legs.

> 환자에게 흉통, 호흡곤란 또는 다리 부종과 같은 합병증의 징후를 지속적으로 관찰하는 것이 중요하다고 교육합니다.

What to say:
↪ "Keep an eye on your symptoms. If you start to feel worse, especially with sudden shortness of breath, chest pain, or significant swelling in your legs, seek immediate medical attention."

> "증상을 주의 깊게 살펴봐 주세요. 갑작스러운 호흡곤란, 흉통 또는 다리의 심한 부종이 나타나면 즉시 의료진에게 연락하시거나 병원을 방문하세요."

Step 6: Documentation and Reporting

6.1 Document the Findings and Patient Response
↪ Record the findings of your DVT and PE assessment, including any positive signs (e.g., swelling, redness, pain, shortness of breath, oxygen saturation, lung auscultation).

Example Documentation:
↪ "Patient assessed for DVT and PE. Right leg showed signs of swelling, tenderness, and warmth, suggestive of possible DVT. O2 saturation measured at 94%, no abnormal breath sounds on auscultation. Patient reports mild shortness of breath. Monitoring and follow-up recommended."

6.2 Report Any Abnormal Findings

- If any red flags are identified (e.g., signs of PE, DVT), report these findings to the medical team immediately for further investigation.

What to say:

- "I've documented my findings and will report any concerning signs to the medical team for further evaluation."

연습 Scenario 1:

Vaginal Packing removal for Patient with ongoing Bleeding

* Time: 10 minutes
* Setting: Gynaecology Surgical Ward
* Situation: Per Vaginal Packing Removal for Patient with Bleeding Symptoms

Example Scenario Description:

You are a registered nurse working in a medical ward. Your patient, Mrs. Linda Roberts, is a 45-year-old female who recently underwent a Hysterectomy that required vaginal packing to control post-operative bleeding. The packing needs to be removed now, and the patient has been showing signs of ongoing bleeding. You must remove the packing safely, assess the site for further bleeding, and monitor the patient's overall condition.

Your task is to safely remove the per vaginal packing, assess the patient's bleeding status, and ensure proper physiological evaluation to determine if further interventions are necessary.

Candidate Instructions:

Step 1: Patient Communication and Preparation

1.1 Introduce Yourself and Confirm Identity
- Knock on the door, greet the patient, and check their identity.

What to say:
- "Good morning, Mrs. Roberts. My name is [Your Name], and I am your nurse today. Could you please confirm your full name and date of birth? Thank you."

1.2 Explain the Procedure and Obtain Consent
- Explain the purpose of packing removal, potential discomfort, and the importance of monitoring bleeding.

What to say:
- "I'm going to remove the vaginal packing to assess the bleeding status. You may feel some pressure during the procedure, but it shouldn't be painful. I will monitor you closely afterward. Do you have any questions before we begin?"

: Obtain verbal consent before proceeding.

1.3 Ensure Patient Comfort and Positioning
- Ensure the patient is in a comfortable position with proper access to the vaginal area. A reclining or semi-reclining position is usually preferred.

What to say:
- "Please lie back in a comfortable position with your knees slightly bent. Let me know if you feel any discomfort during the procedure."

Step 2: Equipment Preparation and Aseptic Technique
2.1 Gather Required Equipment
- Sterile gloves
- Sterile drapes
- Vaginal speculum (if required)
- Sterile gauze
- Absorbent pad
- Sterile scissors or packing removal tool
- Lubricant
- Sharps container for disposal
- Biohazard bag (for used materials)
  : Ensure all equipment is sterile and ready for use.

2.2 Perform Hand Hygiene and Wear PPE
- Wash hands thoroughly and wear sterile gloves. If necessary, wear an apron and mask.

What to say:
- "I am now washing my hands and wearing gloves to ensure that everything is sterile during this procedure."

Step 3: Per Vaginal Packing Removal

3.1 Inspect the Packing Site for Bleeding and Infection
➢ Before removing the packing, inspect the vaginal area for any signs of active bleeding, infection, or unusual discharge. Check if the packing is fully saturated with blood or if the bleeding seems excessive.

What to say:
➢ "I'm going to inspect the area to check for any signs of infection or excessive bleeding before I remove the packing."

3.2 Remove the Packing Gently
➢ Using sterile technique, gently remove the packing by slowly pulling it out, ensuring not to cause further trauma to the tissue. Be cautious of excessive bleeding during the removal.

What to say:
➢ "I'll carefully remove the packing now. Please let me know if you feel any discomfort."

3.3 Control Bleeding During Removal
➢ If the patient begins to bleed more heavily during the removal, apply gentle pressure with sterile gauze to control the bleeding.

What to say:
➢ "I see some bleeding now, so I'm applying gentle pressure to help stop it."

Step 4: Physiological Assessment and Monitoring

4.1 Monitor Vital Signs
⤳ Take the patient's vital signs, including blood pressure, heart rate, and respiratory rate. A sudden drop in blood pressure or a rapid heart rate could indicate excessive bleeding or shock.

What to say:
⤳ "I'm going to check your vital signs now to make sure you're stable after the procedure."

4.2 Assess for Hypovolemic Shock Symptoms
⤳ Monitor for signs of hypovolemic shock such as pallor, dizziness, weakness, and confusion. These signs may indicate that the patient is losing too much blood.

What to say:
⤳ "Let me know if you feel lightheaded, dizzy, or unusually weak, as these can be signs of blood loss."

4.3 Assess the Bleeding Site
⤳ Assess the vaginal area for continued bleeding after packing removal. If bleeding is excessive, apply further pressure or use additional absorbent material.

What to say:
⤳ "I'm checking the bleeding site now. If the bleeding continues, we may need to apply additional pressure or use other measures."

Step 5: Post-Procedure Care and Patient Education

5.1 Dispose of Used Equipment Properly
↳ Dispose of used materials (e.g., gloves, gauze, packing) in the appropriate biohazard bag or sharps container.

What to say:
↳ "I'm disposing of the used materials now in the appropriate containers."

5.2 Monitor for Further Bleeding
↳ Monitor the patient for any signs of re-bleeding. If bleeding continues or worsens, notify the medical team immediately.

What to say:
↳ "Please let me know immediately if you notice any further bleeding or if you feel unwell in any way."

5.3 Provide Patient Education on Bleeding Management
↳ Explain the importance of monitoring for excessive bleeding at home and when to seek immediate medical attention.

What to say:
↳ "After this procedure, it's important to monitor for signs of bleeding. If the bleeding increases or if you experience dizziness or weakness, contact us right away."

Step 6: Documentation and Reporting

6.1 Document the Procedure and Patient Response

⤳ Record the time and date of the packing removal. Document the condition of the vaginal site (bleeding, infection, etc.) and the patient's response to the procedure.

Example Documentation:

⤳ "Per vaginal packing removed for patient Mrs. Linda Roberts. Site inspected for bleeding, moderate bleeding noted upon removal, no signs of infection. Bleeding controlled with pressure. Patient stable post-procedure, vital signs stable, and no further complications observed."

6.2 Report Any Abnormal Findings

⤳ If there is any excessive bleeding or signs of infection or complications, report these findings to the medical team immediately.

What to say:

⤳ "I've documented the procedure and the patient's response. Any excessive bleeding will be reported to the medical team for further evaluation."

④ 전문적인 답변

Station Four: Professional Responsibility

* Time: 10 minutes
* Setting: General practice clinic
* Patient: Mr. John Smith, 55 years old
* Situation: Medication Administration and Error Reporting

✍ Example Example Scenario Description:

You are a nurse working in a busy medical ward, responsible for administering medications to multiple patients. While preparing to administer a prescribed medication to one of your patients, you accidentally misread the medication order and administer the wrong dose. Upon realizing the mistake, you feel a sense of urgency to ensure the patient's safety and correct the error promptly.

당신은 바쁜 병동에서 여러 명의 환자에게 약물을 투여하는 일을 맡고 있는 간호사입니다. 한 환자에게 처방된 약물을 투여하기 위해 준비하던 중, 약물 처방을 잘못 읽고 잘못된 용량을 투여하게 됩니다. 실수를 깨닫자마자 당신은 환자의 안전을 보장하고 오류를 신속하게 수정해야 한다는 촉박감이 듭니다.

✒ Candidate instructions:

1. Acknowledge the Error

As soon as you realize the error, it's important to verbally acknowledge that a mistake has occurred. Be open, honest, and calm when explaining the situation. It's crucial to immediately recognize the mistake, as this sets the tone for the next steps in the process. Be sure to reassure the patient that you're taking the necessary actions to correct it promptly.

> 실수를 깨닫자마자 오류가 발생했음을 인정하는 것이 중요합니다. 상황을 설명할 때는 솔직하고 차분하게 설명해야 합니다. 실수를 즉시 인식하는 것이 중요하며, 이는 이후 절차의 진행 방향을 설정하는 데 큰 역할을 합니다. 환자에게는 필요한 조치를 신속하게 취하고 있음을 확신시켜 주어야 합니다.

What to say:

"I've just realized that I have administered the incorrect dose of your medication. I want to acknowledge this mistake right away and take immediate action to correct it. Your safety is my top priority, and I will make sure everything is handled carefully from here on out."

> "저는 지금 환자분께 잘못된 용량의 약물을 투여했다는 것을 깨달았습니다. 제 실수를 인정하고, 즉각적인 조치를 취하겠습니다. 환자분의 안전이 최우선이며, 앞으로 모든 과정이 신중하게 처리되도록 하겠습니다."

2. Patient Safety

Once you've acknowledged the error, your next priority is the patient's safety. Immediately assess the patient for any signs of adverse reactions or discomfort that may have resulted from the medication error. This includes checking vital signs such as blood pressure, heart rate, oxygen saturation, and respiratory rate. Be alert for any symptoms like shortness of breath, dizziness, or unusual pain. It's essential to monitor the patient closely for any changes and offer reassurance while doing so.

> 오류를 인정한 후, 다음으로 가장 중요한 것은 환자의 안전입니다. 약물 오류로 인해 발생할 수 있는 부작용이나 불편함의 징후를 즉시 사정해야 합니다. 이는 혈압, 심박수, 산소 포화도, 호흡수와 같은 생명징후를 확인하는 것을 포함합니다. 호흡곤란, 어지러움, 또는 이상한 통증과 같은 증상에 주의해야 합니다. 환자의 상태 변화를 면밀히 모니터링하고, 그 과정에서 환자에게 안심을 주는 것이 중요합니다.

What to say:

"I'm going to monitor your condition closely right now. I'll check your blood pressure, heart rate, and breathing to make sure you're not experiencing any adverse reactions. If you feel any discomfort, pain, or notice anything unusual, please let me know immediately."

> "저는 지금 지금부터 당신의 상태를 면밀히 모니터링할 것입니다. 혈압, 심박수, 호흡을 확인하여 부작용이 없으신지 점검하겠습니다. 불편함이나 통증을 느끼거나 이상한 점이 있으면 즉시 말씀해 주세요."

3. Reporting the Error

Following hospital protocol is critical in this situation. As soon as you have realised error, report the error to your supervisor or the appropriate authority within the healthcare system. Make sure you follow the steps outlined in the protocol for medication errors, which typically include documentation and notification of the healthcare team. Ensure that the error is properly recorded in the patient's medical chart, which helps maintain accurate records for both legal and clinical purposes.

> 이 상황에서는 병원 프로토콜을 따르는 것이 매우 중요합니다. 약물오류를 발견하는 순간 오류를 상급자나 의료 시스템 내의 적절한 담당자에게 보고해야 합니다. 약물 오류에 대한 프로토콜에 따라 필요한 절차를 따르도록 합니다. 이는 일반적으로 문서화와 의료 팀에 대한 통지를 포함하며, 환자의 의무기록에 오류가 정확히 기록되도록 해야 합니다. 이는 법적 및 임상적인 목적을 위해 정확한 기록을 유지하는 데 도움이 됩니다.

What to say:

"I will report this medication error to my supervisor immediately. I'll follow the necessary protocol to document the situation correctly, and I'll make sure all relevant information is recorded in your medical record so that we can address this thoroughly."

> "약물 오류를 즉시 제 상사에게 보고하겠습니다. 상황을 정확히 문서화하기 위해 필요한 프로토콜을 따를 것이며, 모든 관련 정보가 귀하의 의무기록에 기록되도록 하여 이 문제를 철저히 해결할 수 있도록 하겠습니다."

4. Communication

Clear and compassionate communication is key when dealing with the patient and their family. Take the time to explain what happened, why it happened, and what steps you are taking to address the situation. Being transparent helps to build trust, and addressing any concerns the patient or family may have is essential. Keep the lines of communication open throughout the process, updating them regularly and offering support. This also includes answering any questions they might have and providing reassurance that their safety is the primary concern.

> 환자와 가족을 대할 때는 명확하고 연민심을 가진 마음으로 의사소통을 하는 것이 중요합니다. 무슨 일이 일어났는지, 왜 일어났는지, 그리고 이를 해결하기 위해 어떤 조치를 취하고 있는지 설명하는 데 시간을 투자해야 합니다. 투명하게 소통하는 것은 신뢰를 쌓는 데 도움이 되며, 환자나 가족이 가질 수 있는 우려를 해결하는 것이 필수적입니다. 이 과정 내내 의사소통의 창을 열어 두고, 정기적으로 업데이트를 제공하며 지원을 아끼지 않아야 합니다. 또한, 그들의 질문에 답하고, 환자의 안전이 최우선임을 확신시켜 주는 것도 포함됩니다.

What to say:

"I apologize for the mistake I made in administering your medication. I understand how this can be concerning. I'm taking immediate steps to ensure your safety, including monitoring you closely for any reactions. If you have any questions or concerns, please don't hesitate to ask. I will keep you updated as we monitor your condition."

> "제가 약물을 투여하는 과정에서 실수를 한 점에 대해 사과드립니다. 이로 인해 걱정이 되실 수 있다는 것을 이해합니다. 환자님의 안전을 보장하기 위해 즉시 조치를 취하고 있으며, 반응을 면밀히 모니터링하고 있습니다. 질문이나 우려 사항이 있으시면 언제든지 말씀해 주세요. 환자님의 상태를 모니터링하면서 계속해서 업데이트를 드리겠습니다."

5. Reflective Practice

After addressing the immediate needs of the patient, take the time to reflect on the error and what led to it. Reflective practice involves understanding the circumstances that contributed to the mistake and considering ways to prevent it from happening again. Identify any factors that may have led to the error, whether it was a distraction, a miscommunication, or a procedural issue. It's important to adopt strategies, such as double-checking medications or seeking guidance when unsure, to prevent future errors. Engage in discussions with colleagues to learn from the situation and improve the overall process.

> 환자에게 필요한 즉각적인 사항들을 해결한 후, 실수와 그 원인에 대해 반성하는 시간을 가지는 것이 중요합니다. 이는 실수가 발생한 상황을 이해하고, 그것이 다시 발생하지 않도록 예방할 방법을 고려하는 과정입니다. 실수를 초래한 요인이 무엇이었는지, 예를 들어 방해 요소, 의사소통의 오류, 또는 절차상의 문제 등을 파악해야 합니다. 향후 오류를 방지하기 위해 약물 투여 전에 이중 확인을 하거나 불확실할 때 동료의 도움을 받는 것과 같은 전략을 세우는 것이 중요합니다. 동료들과 이 상황에 대해 논의하고 배우고, 전반적인 프로세스를 개선하는 데 기여해야 합니다.

What to say:

"I'll be reflecting on this situation to understand what caused the error. I know it's crucial to double-check medication orders and doses, and I will ensure that I always do so in the future. I'll also consider seeking assistance from a colleague when I have any doubts to make sure we maintain the highest standards of care. I'll work on improving my own practice to ensure this doesn't happen again."

"저는 이번 상황에 대해 반성하며 실수가 발생한 원인을 이해하려고 노력할 것입니다. 약물 처방과 용량을 이중 확인하는 것이 매우 중요하다는 것을 알고 있으며, 앞으로 항상 그렇게 하도록 할 것입니다. 또한, 불확실할 때는 동료에게 도움을 요청하여 우리가 최고의 케어 를 제공하고 그를 유지할 수 있도록 하겠습니다. 이번 일이 다시 발생하지 않도록 저의 practice을 개선해 나가겠습니다."

연습 Scenario 1:
Handling Confidential Information

* Time: 10 minutes
* Setting: Outpatient Clinic
* Situation: A colleague accidentally disclosed a patient's private information in a public area, resulting in a breach of confidentiality

✏ Example Scenario Description:

You are a registered nurse working in an outpatient clinic. While reviewing patient charts at the nursing station, you overhear a colleague discussing a patient's private medical information in a public area where other patients and staff can hear. Your task is to manage the situation professionally, ensuring patient confidentiality is upheld and taking appropriate actions.

✍ Candidate Instructions:

1. Immediate Action
- Politely interrupt the conversation to remind your colleague that discussing patient information in public areas is not appropriate.
- Ensure that the conversation is moved to a private area immediately to prevent further exposure of sensitive information.

What to say to the colleague:
- "Excuse me, I understand that you're trying to discuss the patient's information, but we need to make sure all conversations about patients are kept private. Let's step into a private area so we can continue this discussion."

2. Educating the Colleague
- After moving to a private space, explain the importance of maintaining patient confidentiality, emphasizing the ethical and legal implications of breaches.
- Discuss the potential consequences, such as compromising patient trust, legal repercussions, and damage to the clinic's reputation.

What to say to the colleague:
- "I just wanted to remind you about the importance of keeping patient information confidential. Discussing

medical details in public areas, even unintentionally, can result in a breach of confidentiality. This can undermine trust with our patients and lead to serious legal consequences for us as healthcare professionals. Let's make sure we're always mindful of where we're discussing patient information."

3. Patient Advocacy

- If you suspect or know that the patient overheard the conversation, approach them in a calm and empathetic manner.
- Reassure them that their privacy is a priority and that steps are being taken to address the situation.

What to say to the patient:
- "I would like to apologize for what you may have overheard. Patient privacy is extremely important to us, and I want to reassure you that this is being addressed immediately. If you have any concerns or questions, please feel free to ask me, and I'll do my best to address them."

4. Reporting and Documentation

- Document the incident according to the clinic's policy. Include details of the situation, the actions taken to address the breach, and any communication with the patient.

↳ Report the incident to your supervisor or manager as required by the clinic's policies to ensure proper handling and investigation of the breach.

What to document:
↳ "On [Date], I overheard a colleague discussing confidential patient information in a public area. The conversation was immediately interrupted, and the colleague was reminded of the importance of maintaining confidentiality. I spoke with the patient to reassure them of our commitment to privacy. The incident has been reported to the supervisor per clinic policy."

What to say to your supervisor:
↳ "I need to report an incident where a colleague inadvertently discussed a patient's confidential information in a public space. I addressed the situation immediately and reassured the patient. I wanted to make sure you are informed about the breach and the steps I've taken."

❺ 응급상황 관리

Station Five: Emergency management

* **Time: 10 minutes**
* **Setting: Outpatient clinic**
* **Patient: Mr. John Smith, 55 years old**
* **Situation: A patient who received an antibiotic injection and is now presenting with severe allergic reactions.(Sudden onset of difficulty breathing, swelling of the face and lips, and a rapid, weak pulse)**

✎ Example Example Scenario Description:

You are working as a nurse in an outpatient clinic. A patient, who was recently administered an antibiotic injection, suddenly developed severe allergic symptoms, including difficulty breathing, swelling of the face and lips, and a rapid, weak pulse. The patient is visibly anxious and distressed.

> 당신은 외래 진료소에서 간호사로 일하고 있습니다. 최근 항생제 주사를 맞은 환자가 갑자기 심한 알레르기 증상, 즉 호흡 곤란, 얼굴과 입술의 부기, 빠르고 약한 맥박을 보이며, 환자는 명백히 불안하고 고통스러워 보입니다.

Candidate instructions:

1. Recognize the Signs and Symptoms of Anaphylactic Shock:

What the candidate can say:

↘ To the patient: "I can see that you're having trouble breathing, and your face is swelling. These signs suggest you may be having an allergic reaction to the medication. I'm going to help you right away."

> 환자분, 호흡이 어려워지고 얼굴이 부풀어 오른 것을 보니, 약물에 알레르기 반응을 일으키고 있을 수 있습니다. 지금 바로 도와드리겠습니다.

Rationale:

↘ Anaphylactic shock is a life-threatening allergic reaction that requires immediate intervention. The candidate must recognize the signs and symptoms, which include respiratory distress, swelling of the face and lips, and a rapid, weak pulse. Early identification is critical to initiate the proper course of treatment.

> 아나필락틱 쇼크는 즉각적인 개입이 필요한 생명을 위협하는 알레르기 반응입니다. Candidate는 호흡 곤란, 얼굴과 입술의 부기, 빠르고 약한 맥박을 포함한 징후와 증상을 인지해야 합니다. 조기 식별은 적절한 치료 과정을 시작하는 데 매우 중요합니다.

2. Administer the Appropriate Emergency Medications(e.g., Epinephrine):

What the candidate can say:

↪ To the patient: "I am going to give you an injection of epinephrine to help reverse this allergic reaction. This will help you breathe more easily and reduce the swelling."

> 알레르기 반응을 역전시키기 위해 에피네프린 주사를 드리겠습니다. 이것이 호흡을 더 쉽게 하고 부기를 줄이는 데 도움이 될 것입니다.

Rationale:

↪ Epinephrine is the first-line treatment for anaphylactic shock. It works by constricting blood vessels to counteract hypotension, relaxing the muscles around the airways to alleviate breathing difficulty, and reducing swelling. Administering this medication quickly can prevent fatal outcomes.

> 에피네프린은 아나필락틱 쇼크의 1차 치료법입니다. 이 약물은 혈관을 수축시켜 저혈압을 예방하고, 기도 주변의 근육을 이완시켜 호흡 곤란을 완화하며, 부기를 줄이는 역할을 합니다. 이 약물을 빠르게 투여하면 치명적인 결과를 예방할 수 있습니다.

3. Implement Airway Management Techniques:

What the candidate can say:

↪ To the patient: "I'm going to help you breathe more easily. Try to stay calm. I will support your breathing as we get you the necessary treatment."

> 호흡을 더 쉽게 도와드리겠습니다. 차분하게 유지하세요. 필요한 치료를 받으실 수 있도록 호흡완화를 도와드리겠습니다.

Rationale:

- Maintaining a clear airway is crucial in patients experiencing anaphylactic shock, as airway constriction and oedema can impede breathing. Elevating the head of the bed can aid in easier breathing, and supplemental oxygen may be required if the patient's oxygen saturation is low.

> 아나필락틱 쇼크를 경험하는 환자에게는 기도를 유지하는 것이 매우 중요합니다. 기도 수축과 부기가 호흡을 방해할 수 있기 때문입니다. 침대 머리를 높이면 호흡이 더 쉬워질 수 있으며, 환자의 산소 포화도가 낮으면 추가 산소 공급이 필요할 수 있습니다.

4. Monitor Vital Signs and Prepare for Possible Advanced Interventions:

What the candidate can say:

- To the patient: "I'm going to monitor your vital signs closely to make sure you're stabilizing, and I'll let the doctor know if we need further intervention."

> 환자분, 저는 환자분이 안정되고 있는지 확인하기 위해 활력징후를 면밀히 모니터링할 것이며, 추가 처치가 필요하면 의사에게 보고하겠습니다.

Rationale:

- Monitoring vital signs(heart rate, blood pressure, respiratory rate, oxygen saturation) is essential for assessing the effectiveness of the initial interventions and ensuring that the patient is stabilizing. If the patient's condition worsens, further interventions such as fluid resuscitation, additional epinephrine doses, or intubation may be needed.

> 활력징후(심박수, 혈압, 호흡수, 산소 포화도)를 모니터링하는 것은 초기 처치의 효과를 평가하고 환자가 안정되고 있는지 확인하는 데 필수적입니다. 환자의 상태가 악화되면, 수액 투여, 추가적인 에피네프린 투여 또는 기관내 삽관과 같은 추가 처치가 필요할 수 있습니다.

5. Communicate with the Healthcare Team for Urgent Support:

What the candidate can say:

↪ To the patient(while communicating with the team): "I've given you epinephrine, and I'm monitoring you closely. I'm also calling the doctor and the emergency team to come in right away, just in case you need further treatment."

> 저는 에피네프린을 드렸고, 환자분을 면밀히 모니터링하고 있습니다. 또한, 추가 치료가 필요할 경우를 대비해 의사와 응급팀에 연락하고 있습니다.

↪ To the healthcare team: "We have a patient with anaphylactic shock. I've administered epinephrine and am monitoring their vital signs. Could you please assist with further management and any necessary interventions?"

> 아나필락틱 쇼크를 겪고 있는 환자가 있습니다. 에피네프린을 투여하고 활력징후를 모니터링하고 있습니다. 추가 처치 및 필요한 중재에 대해 도와주실 수 있으신가요?"

Rationale:

↪ Clear and effective communication with the healthcare team is crucial to ensure timely and coordinated care. The candidate must promptly inform the doctor and other relevant team members, such as an emergency response team, so they can intervene as needed.

> 의료팀과의 명확하고 효과적인 소통은 신속하고 협력적인 치료를 보장하는 데 중요합니다. 후보자는 의사와 응급 대응팀과 같은 관련 팀원들에게 즉시 상황을 알리고, 필요시 그들이 개입할 수 있도록 해야 합니다.

6. Document the Incident:

Rationale:

↪ Documentation ensures legal and clinical accountability. The nurse must record the sequence of events, including symptoms, interventions, and any communications with other healthcare professionals. This will be critical for ongoing patient care and potential future legal or clinical reviews.

✱ Example

Date/Time: [date and time of the event]
Patient: Mr. [patient name]
DOB: [patient's date of birth]
Location: Outpatient Clinic

Subjective:
- Patient presents with complaints of difficulty breathing, facial swelling, and a weak, rapid pulse after receiving an antibiotic injection. The patient appears anxious and visibly distressed.

Objective:
- Vital signs:
  - HR, BP, RR, O2 Sat, Temperature
- Physical Exam Findings:
  - Swelling noted on the face and lips.
  - Respiratory distress observed.
  - Rapid and weak pulse.
  - Patient appears anxious and is struggling to breathe.

Assessment:
- Clinical signs and symptoms consistent with anaphylactic shock following antibiotic administration. Immediate intervention is required to manage the patient's airway, breathing, and circulation.

Plan/Intervention:
1.1 Administered epinephrine 0.5mg IM as per anaphylactic shock protocol.

1.2 Positioned the patient with the head elevated to assist with breathing.

1.3 Administered oxygen via [insert method] at [insert flow rate].

1.4 Vital signs are being monitored every [insert interval] to assess response to treatment.

1.5 Notified the doctor and emergency team regarding the patient's condition for further support.

1.6 Documented patient's response to the interventions and ongoing monitoring.

↳ Patient Response:

- After epinephrine injection, patient's respiratory effort slightly improved. Facial swelling continues but is less pronounced. Pulse remains weak but less rapid. Patient reports some relief from breathing difficulty but remains anxious.

↳ Follow-up/Plan:

- Continue to monitor vital signs and symptoms closely.
- Emergency team and doctor to reassess patient for possible further treatment.
- Continue to monitor for any signs of deterioration or worsening condition.

Signature:

[nurse's name and title]

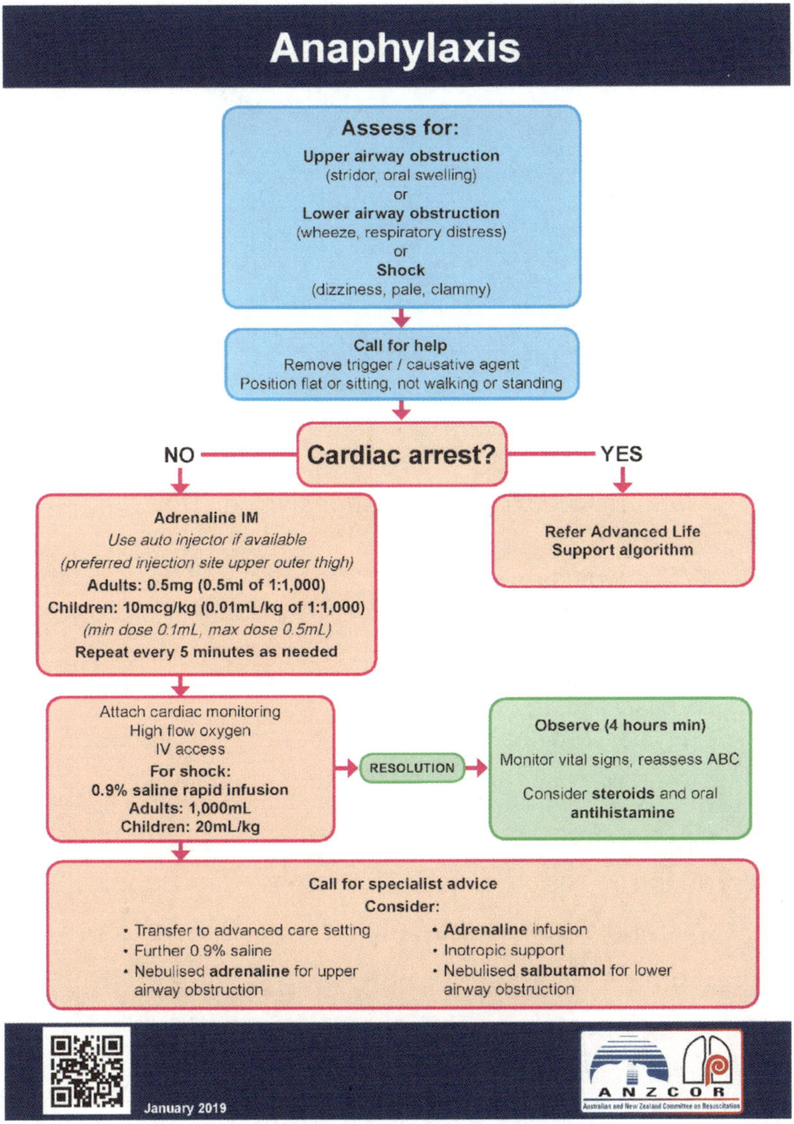

Anaphylaxis

Assess for:
Upper airway obstruction
(stridor, oral swelling)
or
Lower airway obstruction
(wheeze, respiratory distress)
or
Shock
(dizziness, pale, clammy)

Call for help
Remove trigger / causative agent
Position flat or sitting, not walking or standing

Cardiac arrest?

NO →

Adrenaline IM
Use auto injector if available
(preferred injection site upper outer thigh)
Adults: 0.5mg (0.5ml of 1:1,000)
Children: 10mcg/kg (0.01mL/kg of 1:1,000)
(min dose 0.1mL, max dose 0.5mL)
Repeat every 5 minutes as needed

YES →

Refer Advanced Life Support algorithm

Attach cardiac monitoring
High flow oxygen
IV access
For shock:
0.9% saline rapid infusion
Adults: 1,000mL
Children: 20mL/kg

→ **RESOLUTION** →

Observe (4 hours min)

Monitor vital signs, reassess ABC

Consider **steroids** and oral **antihistamine**

Call for specialist advice
Consider:
- Transfer to advanced care setting
- Further 0.9% saline
- Nebulised **adrenaline** for upper airway obstruction
- **Adrenaline** infusion
- Inotropic support
- Nebulised **salbutamol** for lower airway obstruction

January 2019

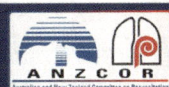

연습 Scenario 1:
Cardiac Arrest

* Time: 10 minutes
* Setting: Hospital Corridor
* Patient: 65-year-old male
* Presenting Complaint: Unresponsive, no detectable pulse

✎ Example Scenario Description:

A 65-year-old male patient suddenly collapses in the hospital corridor. On arrival, you find the patient lying on the ground, unresponsive, with no detectable pulse. Immediate intervention is required to initiate Basic Life Support(BLS) protocols and stabilize the patient. Your task is to provide rapid, effective resuscitation efforts, utilize available emergency equipment, and coordinate with the healthcare team for advanced care.

The situation demands prioritization of tasks, clear communication, and the ability to remain calm under pressure. You must demonstrate competency in performing CPR, using an Automated External Defibrillator(AED), and managing the airway. Effective teamwork and proper documentation of the incident are critical components of this scenario.

Candidate Instructions:

1. Initiate Basic Life Support(BLS):

1.1 Assess the patient's responsiveness and call for help immediately.

- "Can you hear me? Are you okay?"(Tap the patient's shoulders to check for a response.)
- "I need help here! Call for emergency support and bring the crash cart!"

1.2 Begin chest compressions at the appropriate depth and rate(30 compressions to 2 rescue breaths).

- "I'm starting chest compressions now, pushing hard and fast in the centre of the chest."
- "Make sure we minimize interruptions, keep the compressions effective!"
- Ensure compressions are effective by allowing full chest recoil and minimizing interruptions.
- "Let's rotate compressors every two minutes to prevent fatigue."
- "Ensure full chest recoil between compressions to allow proper circulation."

2. Use the Automated External Defibrillator(AED):

2.1 Retrieve and apply the AED as soon as possible.

- ✈ "Someone gets the AED now!"
- ✈ "I'm placing the pads on the patient's chest, one on the upper right, one on the lower left."

2.2 Follow the AED's voice prompts to assess the need for defibrillation.

- ✈ "Analysing heart rhythm, do not touch the patient!"
- ✈ "Everyone clear! stay back while the AED checks for a shockable rhythm!"

2.3 Deliver the shock if indicated, ensuring everyone is clear of the patient before activating the device.

- ✈ "Shock advised! Everyone, step back, CLEAR!" (After delivering the shock) "Resuming chest compressions immediately!"

3. Manage the Airway:

3.1 Open the airway using the head-tilt chin-lift or jaw-thrust manoeuvre.

- ✈ "The airway is obstructed, I'm performing a head-tilt chin-lift to open it."
- ✈ "If there's a spinal injury suspected, let's use the jaw-thrust manoeuvre instead."

3.2 Use a bag-valve-mask to provide rescue breaths or administer oxygen as needed.

- ✈ "I'm providing two rescue breaths now, ensuring good chest rise with each breath."
- ✈ "Let's attach the oxygen to the bag-valve mask for better oxygenation."

3.3 If equipment is available, prepare to use an airway adjunct such as an oropharyngeal or nasopharyngeal airway.
- "The patient is not maintaining an open airway, I'm inserting an oropharyngeal airway."
- "If there's a gag reflex, we'll use a nasopharyngeal airway instead."

4. Coordinate with the Resuscitation Team:

4.1 Provide a clear and concise handover to the arriving resuscitation team.
- "Patient is unresponsive, found in cardiac arrest. We started CPR at [time]. AED has delivered [number] shocks. Currently in [rhythm]."

4.2 Communicate details of the patient's condition, the time the arrest occurred, and interventions performed.
- "Compressions have been ongoing with minimal interruptions. AED was applied after [time] minutes. No spontaneous circulation detected yet."

4.3 Continue assisting the team as directed.
- "I'll continue compressions unless someone else takes over."
- "I'm ready to assist with medication administration or airway management."

5. Document the Event:

5.1 Record the time of the collapse, actions taken, and the patient's response to interventions.

↳ "Documenting the exact time of collapse and the start of CPR."

↳ "Noting each intervention performed, including the number of shocks delivered."

5.2 Note any use of the AED, including the number of shocks delivered and the rhythm detected.

↳ "AED analysis showed [rhythm] before delivering [number] of shocks."

↳ "Patient remained pulseless, continuous resuscitation efforts documented."

5.3 Ensure that all details are accurately documented in the patient's record for legal and clinical purposes.

↳ "Completing the resuscitation report to ensure an accurate and detailed record."

↳ "All information will be included in the patient's file for legal and medical review."

https://www.anzcor.org/

Advanced Life Support for Adults

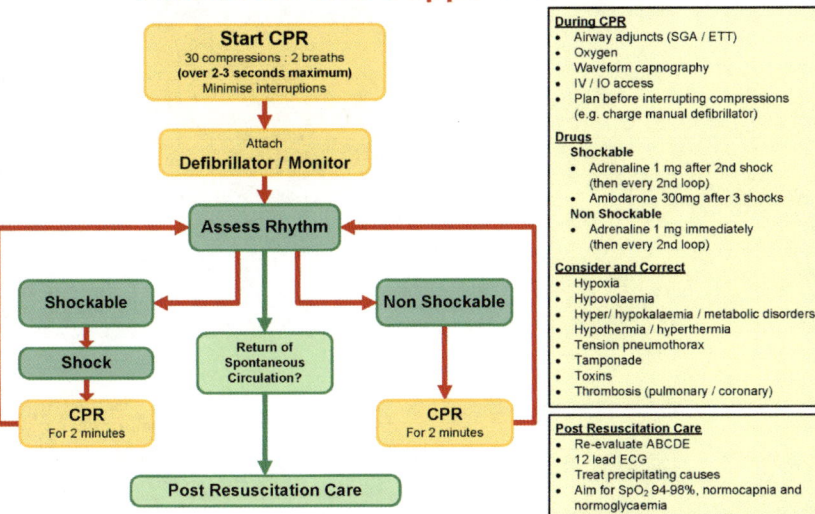

6 임상 술기(상처드레싱 교환)

Clinical Skills

* Time: 10 minutes
* Setting: Medical Ward
* Situation: Indwelling Catheter Insertion(IDC) for Urinary Retention.

✎ Example Example Scenario Description:

You are a registered nurse working in a medical ward. Your patient, Mr. James Anderson, a 72-year-old male, has been experiencing acute urinary retention secondary to benign prostatic hyperplasia(BPH). He has a distended bladder, complains of severe lower abdominal discomfort, and has not passed urine in over eight hours despite hydration. His doctor has ordered an indwelling urinary catheter(IDC) to relieve the retention. Your task is to explain the procedure to the patient, prepare for catheterization, insert the catheter safely using aseptic technique, ensure proper aftercare, and document the procedure appropriately.

당신은 Medical병동에서 근무하는 간호사입니다. 담당 환자, James Anderson씨(72세 남성)는 양성 전립선 비대증(BPH)으로 인한 급성 배뇨 정체를 경험하고 있습니다. 그는 방광 팽만감을 느끼고 심한 하복부 불편감을 호소하며, 수분 보충에도 불구하고 8시간 이상 소변을 보지 못했습니다. 그의 의사는 배뇨 정체를 해소하기 위해 도뇨관(IDC)을 삽입하도록 지시하였습니다. Candidate로써 당신은 환자에게 시술 절차를 설명하고, 도뇨관 삽입을 위한 준비를 하며, 무균 기술을 사용하여 도뇨관을 안전하게 삽입하고, 적절한 시술 후 관리 및 기록을 작성하는 것입니다.

Candidate Instructions:

Step 1: Patient Communication and Preparation

1.1. Knock on the door, introduce yourself, and confirm patient identity.

> "Hello Mr. Anderson, my name is [Your Name], and I am your nurse today. Can you confirm your full name and date of birth for me?"

노크를 하고, 자신을 소개한 후 환자의 신원을 확인합니다.
"안녕하세요, Anderson 씨. 제 이름은 [본인의 이름]이고, 오늘 당신을 돌볼 간호사입니다. 성함과 생년월일을 확인해 주실 수 있나요?"

1.2. Explain the procedure in simple terms.

> "I understand you have been experiencing some discomfort due to difficulty passing urine. The doctor has prescribed an indwelling urinary catheter, which is a small flexible tube that will be inserted into your bladder to help drain the urine. This will relieve the pressure and discomfort you are feeling. The procedure should only take a few minutes, and I will ensure it is as comfortable as possible for you. Do you have any concerns or questions before we begin?"

절차를 간단한 용어로 설명합니다.
"소변을 보는데 어려움이 있어 불편함을 겪고 계신 것을 이해합니다. 의사 선생님께서 도뇨관을 삽입하라고 처방하셨습니다. 도뇨관은 작은 유연한 튜브로, 이를 방광에 삽입하여 소변을 배출하는 데 도움을 줄 것입니다. 이렇게 하면 현재 느끼고 계신 압박감과 불편함을 해소할 수 있습니다. 시술은 몇 분 정도만 소요되며, 최대한 편안하게 진행되도록 하겠습니다. 시술을 시작하기 전에 궁금한 점이나 걱정되는 사항이 있으신가요?"

1.3. Obtain informed consent.

↪ "If you're happy for us to proceed, I will begin preparing the equipment and ensure everything is done with sterile technique to prevent infection."

동의서를 받습니다.(Organisation에 따라서 Written 이나 Verbal로 받으면 됩니다, 뉴질랜드에서는 특별한 Written consent가 필요하지는 않고 환자 챠트에 기록해주면 됩니다)
"진행해도 괜찮으시다면, 장비를 준비하고 감염 예방을 위해 모든 절차가 무균 기술로 진행되도록 하겠습니다."

1.4. Ensure privacy and comfort.

↪ Close the curtain and door.
↪ Assist the patient into a supine position with legs slightly apart.
↪ Cover the patient with a drape, exposing only the necessary area.

개인 정보 보호 및 편안함을 보장합니다.
- 커튼과 문을 닫습니다.
- 환자가 무릎을 약간 벌린 상태로 평평한 자세가 되도록 도와줍니다.
- 필요한 부위만 노출되도록 커버로 환자를 덮습니다.

Step 2: Equipment Preparation & Aseptic Technique

2.1. Gather equipment:

- Catheter insertion kit(including sterile gloves, drapes, antiseptic solution, lubricating gel, forceps, and catheter)
- Indwelling catheter of appropriate size(usually 14-16Fr for males, 12-14Fr for females)
- Sterile water for balloon inflation(usually 10ml)
- Urine collection bag
- PPE(gloves, gown, and mask if required)

장비 준비:
- 도뇨관 삽입 키트(무균 장갑, 덮개, 소독액, 윤활 젤, 겸자, 도뇨관 포함)
- 적절한 크기의 도뇨관(남성의 경우 보통 14-16Fr, 여성의 경우 12-14Fr)
- 풍선 팽창을 위한 무균 생리식염수(보통 10ml)
- 소변 수집 백
- PPE(장갑, 가운, 필요 시 마스크)

2.2. Perform hand hygiene and put on PPE.

- Open the catheterization kit using sterile technique.
- Wear sterile gloves and maintain aseptic technique throughout.

손 위생을 수행하고 PPE를 착용합니다.
- 도뇨관 삽입 키트를 무균 기술로 엽니다.
- 무균 장갑을 착용하고 시술 내내 무균 기술을 유지합니다.

2.3. Perineal Cleansing and Preparation

⤳ Male patient:
- Retract the foreskin(if uncircumcised) and hold the penis at a 90-degree angle.
- Cleanse the meatus with antiseptic solution from the urethral opening outward in a circular motion.
- Apply sterile lubricating gel to the catheter tip.

⤳ Female patient:
- Separate the labia using non-dominant hand.
- Cleanse the urethral opening with antiseptic from top to bottom(front to back).
- Apply sterile lubricating gel to the catheter tip.

회음 부위 세정 및 준비
- 남성 환자(** 남성환자의 IDC insertion의 경우 뉴질랜드에서는 추가로 트레이닝을 받은후 Procedure를 진행할수 있습니다)
  · 포경 수술을 하지 않은 경우, 음경을 90도 각도로 들어 foreskin을 뒤로 젖힌다.
  · 소독액을 사용하여 요도구를 원을 그리며 요도 개구부에서 바깥쪽으로 세정한다.
  · 도뇨관 끝에 무균 윤활 젤을 바른다.
- 여성 환자:
  · 주로 쓰지 않는 손으로 음순을 벌린다.
  · 소독액을 사용하여 요도 개구부를 위에서 아래로(앞에서 뒤로) 세정한다.
  · 도뇨관 끝에 무균 윤활 젤을 바른다.

Step 3: Catheter Insertion and Urine Drainage

3.1. Insert the catheter using a steady motion:

⤳ "Mr. Anderson, you may feel some pressure or slight discomfort as I insert the catheter. Take slow, deep breaths to help relax."
- Insert the catheter until urine flows into the tube.

- Advance the catheter 2-3 cm further to ensure it is correctly positioned.

> **도뇨관을 일정한 움직임으로 삽입합니다:**
> "Anderson 씨, 도뇨관을 삽입하면서 압박감이나 약간의 불편함을 느끼실 수 있습니다. 천천히 깊게 숨을 쉬며 이완을 도와주세요."
> - 도뇨관을 삽입하여 소변이 튜브로 흐르도록 합니다.
> - 도뇨관을 2-3cm 더 밀어넣어 정확한 위치에 있는지 확인합니다.

↳ "I can see the urine flowing now. I'm just advancing the catheter a little more to ensure it's in the correct position."
  - Inflate the catheter balloon with sterile water to secure placement.
  - Gently pull back slightly until resistance is felt.

↳ "The catheter is now secured in place. I will attach it to the drainage bag, and you should start to feel relief soon."

> "이제 소변이 흐르는 것을 볼 수 있습니다. 도뇨관을 조금 더 밀어넣어 정확히 위치시킬게요."
> - 도뇨관 풍선에 무균 생리식염수로 공기를 넣어 위치를 고정시킵니다.
> - 저항을 느낄 때까지 살짝 뒤로 당깁니다.
> "도뇨관이 이제 고정되었습니다. 배액 백에 연결할 것이며, 곧 불편함이 완화될 것입니다."

Step 4: Post-Insertion Care and Patient Education

4.1. Secure the catheter and ensure proper positioning

- ↳ Attach the drainage bag to the bed below bladder level.
- ↳ Secure the catheter to the patient's thigh to prevent movement.
- ↳ Ensure no kinks or obstructions in the tubing.

> **도뇨관을 고정하고 적절한 위치를 확인합니다.**
> - 배액 백을 방광보다 낮은 침대에 연결합니다.
> - 도뇨관을 환자의 허벅지에 고정하여 움직이지 않도록 합니다.
> - 튜브에 꼬이거나 막힌 부분이 없는지 확인합니다.

4.2. Assess patient response

- ↳ "How are you feeling now, Mr. Anderson? The discomfort should start to subside as your bladder empties."
- ↳ Monitor urine output, color, and consistency.
- ↳ Observe for signs of infection or complications(e.g., bleeding, pain, leakage).

> **환자의 반응을 평가합니다.**
> "지금 기분이 어떠신가요, Anderson 씨? 방광이 비어가면서 불편함이 점차 줄어들 거예요."
> - 소변의 양, 색상 및 일관성을 모니터링합니다.
> - 감염이나 합병증의 징후(예: 출혈, 통증, 누수 등)를 관찰합니다.

4.3. Provide patient education

↳ "This catheter will remain in place as per the doctor's orders. It is important to keep the drainage bag below the bladder level to ensure proper drainage. If you feel any discomfort, pain, or notice cloudy or foul-smelling urine, please let the nursing team know immediately. I will check on you regularly and make sure everything is working properly."

환자 교육을 제공합니다.
"이 도뇨관은 의사의 지시에 따라 계속 유지됩니다. 적절한 배액을 위해 배액 백을 방광보다 낮은 위치에 두는 것이 중요합니다. 불편함, 통증을 느끼거나 소변이 흐릿하거나 악취가 나면 즉시 간호팀에 알려주세요. 저는 정기적으로 확인하고 모든 것이 제대로 작동하는지 확인하겠습니다."

Step 5: Documentation and Reporting

↳ Record the time and date of catheter insertion.
↳ Note the catheter size, type, and amount of balloon inflation.
↳ Document the patient's response and urine output.
↳ Report any abnormal findings to the doctor.

문서화 및 보고
- 도뇨관 삽입 시간과 날짜를 기록합니다.
- 도뇨관 크기, 유형 및 풍선 팽창 양을 기재합니다.
- 환자의 반응과 소변 양을 문서화합니다.
- 비정상적인 소견이 있으면 의사에게 보고합니다.

✳ Study Tips!!

- Practice catheter insertion on mannequins to perfect technique.
- Memorize the step-by-step process to ensure efficiency during timed OSCE exams.
- Familiarize yourself with different catheter types and sizes for male and female patients.
- Understand catheter-related complications(e.g., infections, trauma, blockages) and how to manage them.
- Use ISBAR when escalating concerns about catheterization difficulties.
- Time yourself during practice to ensure completion within the OSCE time limit.

Fig 1. **Inserting a catheter into a female patient**

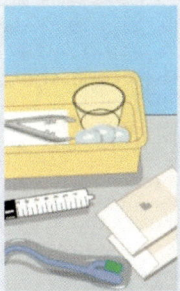

1a. After risk assessment prepare the patient and the equipment

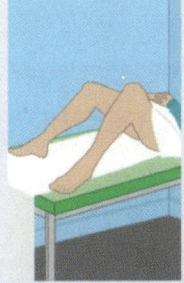

1b. Assist the patient into a supine position with knees bent and feet apart

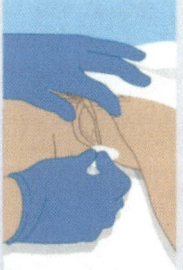

1c. Clean the labia with 0.9% sodium chloride to reduce infection risk

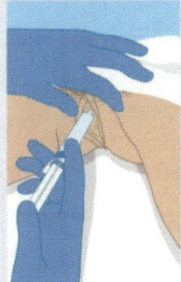

1d. Instill anesthetic or lubricating gel into the urethra to reduce pain and/or urethral trauma

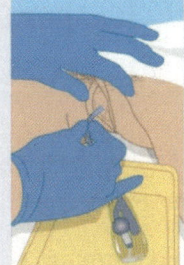

1e. Hold the labia open and insert the catheter into the bladder using your dominant hand

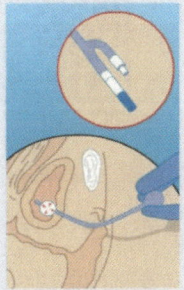

1f. Inflate the balloon and connect to a drainage device or catheter valve

〈Female IDC insertion예시〉

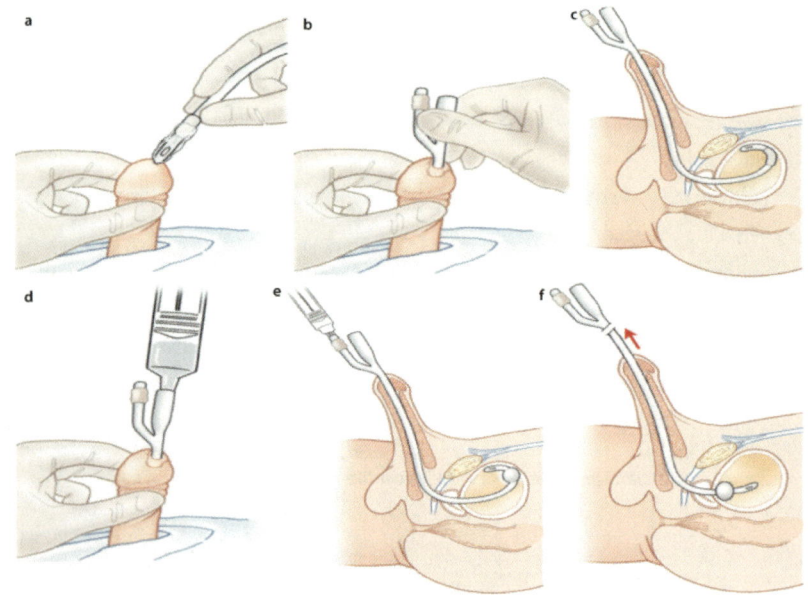

〈Male IDC insertion 예시〉

연습 Scenario 1:
Performing ECG

* Time: 10 minutes
* Setting: Medical Ward
* Situation: Electrocardiogram(ECG) Recording for Cardiac Assessment

🔖 Example Example Scenario Description:

You are a registered nurse working in a medical ward. Your patient, Mr. John Smith, a 65-year-old male, has been experiencing intermittent chest pain and palpitations for the past few hours. His doctor has ordered a 12-lead ECG to assess his cardiac rhythm and detect any potential abnormalities. Your task is to explain the ECG procedure to the patient, prepare the equipment, ensure proper lead placement, obtain a high-quality ECG recording, and document the procedure appropriately.

🖉 Candidate Instructions:

Step 1: Patient Communication and Preparation

1.1. Knock on the door, introduce yourself, and confirm patient identity

- "Hello Mr. Smith, my name is [Your Name], and I am your nurse today. Can you confirm your full name and date of birth for me?"

1.2. Explain the procedure in simple terms

- "The doctor has requested an ECG, which is a quick and painless test to check your heart's electrical activity. Small sticky electrodes will be placed on your chest, arms, and legs, and a machine will record your heart's rhythm. The test will only take a few minutes, and I will ensure your comfort throughout. Do you have any concerns or questions before we begin?"

1.3. Obtain informed consent

- "If you're happy to proceed, I will begin preparing the equipment."

1.4. Ensure privacy and patient comfort

- Close the curtain and door.
- Ask the patient to remove any jewellery or metal objects.
- Assist the patient into a supine position with their arms relaxed at their sides.

- Expose the chest area while maintaining modesty.

Step 2: Equipment Preparation & Skin Preparation

2.1. Gather necessary equipment:
- 12-lead ECG machine.
- Disposable electrodes.
- Skin preparation supplies(e.g., alcohol wipes, razor for hair removal if needed).
- ECG paper and calibration check.

2.2. Perform hand hygiene and wear gloves if needed

2.3. Prepare the skin for electrode placement
- Clean the skin with alcohol wipes to remove oils or lotions.
- Shave excess hair if necessary for proper electrode adhesion.
- Ensure the skin is dry before applying electrodes.

Step 3: ECG Electrode Placement and Lead Connection

3.1. Correctly position the 10 electrodes:

Limb Leads:
- RA(Right Arm): Right wrist or shoulder.
- LA(Left Arm): Left wrist or shoulder.
- RL(Right Leg): Right ankle or lower leg(ground lead).
- LL(Left Leg): Left ankle or lower leg.

Chest(Precordial) Leads:

- V1: 4th intercostal space, right of the sternum.
- V2: 4th intercostal space, left of the sternum.
- V3: Midway between V2 and V4.
- V4: 5th intercostal space, midclavicular line.
- V5: 5th intercostal space, anterior axillary line.
- V6: 5th intercostal space, midaxillary line.

3.2. Attach ECG leads to corresponding electrodes

- Ensure each lead is securely connected.
- Ask the patient to remain still and breathe normally to minimize artifact.

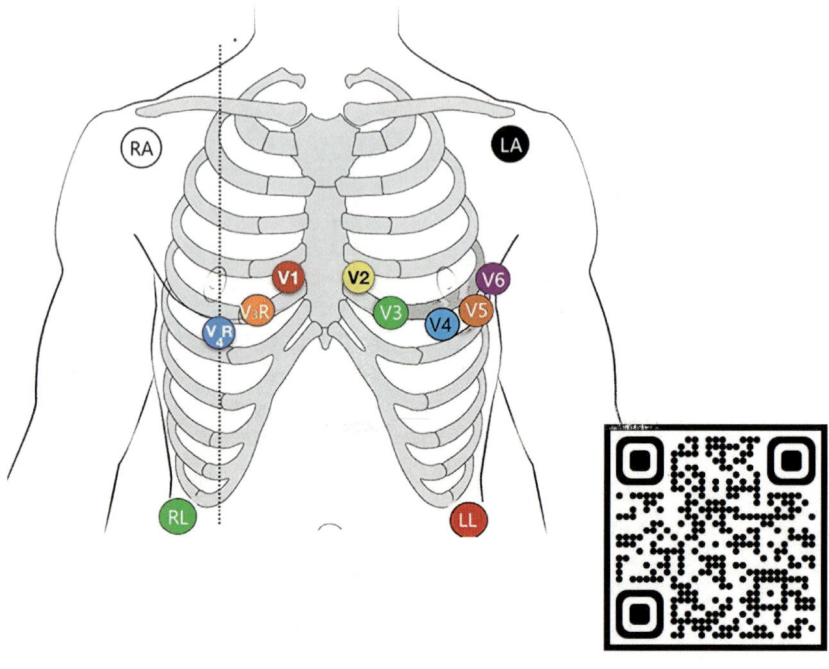

12유도 심전도(ECG)라고 불리는 이유는 총 12개의 서로 다른 유도(lead)를 통해 심장의 전기적 활동을 기록하기 때문입니다.

비록 전극(electrode)은 가슴과 팔다리에 총 10개가 부착되지만, 이 전극들의 조합을 통해 12개의 서로 다른 시점에서 심장의 전기 신호를 분석할 수 있습니다.

* **사지 유도(Limb Leads) - 6개**
- 표준 사지 유도(3개): I, II, III
- 증폭 사지 유도(3개): aVR, aVL, aVF

* **흉부 유도(Precordial Leads) - 6개**
- V1, V2, V3, V4, V5, V6

Step 4: ECG Recording and Quality Check

4.1. Instruct the patient to stay still
↳ "Mr. Smith, please try to relax and stay as still as possible while I record the ECG. This will ensure we get a clear reading."

4.2. Run the ECG recording
↳ Press the appropriate button on the machine to begin recording.
↳ Observe the tracing for any artifacts or irregularities.
↳ Ensure leads are properly connected if interference is noted.
↳ Print and review the ECG strip.

4.3. Assess the ECG quality
- Check for a steady baseline and absence of artifacts.
- Ensure all 12 leads are recorded properly.
- If abnormalities or technical issues arise, reposition electrodes and repeat the test if necessary.

Step 5: Post-Procedure Care and Documentation

5.1. Remove electrodes and clean the patient's skin
- "The ECG is complete. I will now remove the electrodes and make sure you are comfortable."

5.2. Assist the patient with clothing if needed
- Ensure patient privacy is maintained.

5.3. Document the procedure accurately
- Time and date of ECG recording.
- Indication for the ECG(e.g., chest pain, palpitations).
- Any difficulties encountered during the procedure.
- Report abnormal findings to the doctor immediately.

✱ Study Tips!!

- Practice ECG lead placement on mannequins or colleagues.
- Memorize the lead positions for quick and accurate placement.
- Review normal vs. abnormal ECG patterns to understand common findings.
- Time yourself during practice to ensure completion within 10 minutes.
- Understand artifact sources and troubleshooting techniques.
- Use ISBAR when escalating abnormal ECG findings to the medical team.

⑦ 약물 투약

Station Seven: Medication Administration

* Time: 10 minutes
* Setting: Medical Ward
* Situation: A patient is scheduled to receive an oral antihypertensive medication, but the nurse must calculate the correct dose based on the doctor's prescription and the medication available.

🔖 Example Example Scenario Description:

You are a registered nurse on a medical ward. Mr. John Doe, a 58-year-old patient with hypertension, is scheduled to receive his oral antihypertensive medication. The doctor's prescription specifies 25 mg, but the medication available is in 50 mg tablets, requiring dose calculation.

> 당신은 내과병동에서 근무하는 간호사 입니다. 58세의 고혈압 환자인 John Doe씨가 항고혈압 경구약을 복용할 예정인데요, 의사의 처방은 25mg이지만 병동에 있는 약은 50mg정제로 되어 있어 용량 계산이 필요합니다.

Candidate Instructions:

Your task is to ensure the correct dose is administered by performing accurate calculations, confirming the patient's identity, and monitoring for any adverse reactions post-administration. This scenario tests your competency in medication calculation, safe administration, and patient-centered care.

> Candidate의 task 는 정확한 용량을 계산하고 환자의 신원을 확인하며, 약물을 안전하게 투여하고, 투여후 이상 반응을 모니터링 하는 것입니다. 이 시나리오는 약물 계산 능력, 안전한 약물 관리, 환자 중심의 간호능력을 평가합니다.

1. Verify the Medication Order and Patient Identity

- Cross-check the doctor's prescription with the medication available. Use the "7 Rights" of medication administration: right patient, right drug, right dose, right route, right purpose and right time, right documentation. Confirm the patient's identity using at least two identifiers.

> 의사의 처방과 제공된 약물을 교차 확인합니다. 약물 투여의 "7 Rights"을 확인하세요: "올바른 환자, 약물, 용량, 경로, 시간, 목적 기록". 환자의 신원을 확인할때는 적어도 두개의 확인 가능한 identity를 체크합니다.

What to say:

- "Good morning, Mr. Doe. My name is [Name], and I'm your nurse today. Can you please confirm your full name and date of birth for me? Thank you. I see you're scheduled to take your blood pressure medication now, and I'll verify the prescription and calculate your dose before we proceed."

좋은 아침입니다, Mr. Doe. 저는 오늘 당신의 간호사 [이름]입니다. 성함과 생년월일을 확인해 주시겠어요? 감사합니다. 오늘 혈압 약을 복용할 예정이고, 처방을 확인한 후 정확한 용량을 계산하겠습니다.

2. Perform Dose Calculation

↳ Calculate the correct dose based on the prescription and available tablets:
  - Doctor's order: 25 mg.
  - Tablet strength: 50 mg per tablet.
  - Required dose = ½ tablet
    처방된 용량과 제공된 정제를 기반으로 정확한 용량을 계산합니다.
↳ 의사의 처방: 25mg.
↳ 정제 용량: 50mg/정.
↳ 필요한 용량 = 0.5 정

What to say(thinking out loud):

↳ "The prescription is for 25 mg, and the tablets are 50 mg each. That means I'll need to give half a tablet to ensure the correct dose."

처방된 용량은 25mg이고, 정제는 50mg입니다. 따라서 정확한 용량을 위해 반 정제를 투여해야 합니다.

3. Explain the Procedure to the Patient and Obtain Consent

↳ Inform the patient about the medication, its purpose, and any potential side effects. Obtain verbal consent before administering.

약물의 목적과 잠재적 부작용에 대해 환자에게 설명합니다. 투여 전에 구두 동의를 얻습니다.

What to say:

↬ "Mr. Doe, your medication is a blood pressure tablet that helps manage hypertension. Today, your dose is 25 mg, which I've calculated to be half a tablet. This medication might occasionally cause dizziness, so please let me know if you feel unwell after taking it. Are you ok to take it?"

> Mr. Doe, 이 약물은 혈압을 조절하기 위한 약입니다. 오늘의 용량은 25mg이며, 이를 위해 반 정제를 복용해야 합니다. 이 약물은 가끔 어지럼증을 유발할 수 있으니, 복용 후 불편함을 느끼시면 꼭 알려주세요. 복용 괜찮으시겠어요?"

4. Perform Hand Hygiene and Prepare the Medication

↬ Wash your hands thoroughly, prepare the medication in a clean and safe environment, and ensure accuracy in dose preparation.

> 손을 철저히 씻고 깨끗하고 안전한 환경에서 약물을 준비합니다.

What to say(while preparing):

↬ "I'm preparing your dose now, ensuring it's accurate. I'll bring it to you shortly."

> 지금 약을 준비하고 있습니다. 용량이 정확한지 확인 후 바로 가져다 드리겠습니다.

5. Administer the Medication and Monitor the Patient

↬ Provide the medication to the patient and ensure they take it. Observe the patient for any immediate adverse reactions and monitor their blood pressure afterwards.

환자에게 약물을 제공하고 복용을 확인합니다. 즉각적인 이상 반응을 관찰하고 혈압을 포함한 상태를 모니터링합니다.

What to say:
↳ "Here's your medication, Mr. Doe. Please take it with a sip of water. Please let me know if you feel anything unusual.

여기 약이 있습니다, Mr. Doe. 물 한 모금과 함께 드세요. 이상증상이 있으면 바로 알려주세요.

6. Document the Administration
↳ Record the medication administration in the patient's chart, including the dose, time, and any observations.

약물 투여를 포함한 기록을 환자 차트에 정확히 작성합니다.

What to document:
↳ Administered 25 mg of [Medication Name] orally as prescribed. Patient tolerated the medication well, with no immediate adverse reactions noted. Blood pressure and other vitals will be monitored as per protocol.

처방대로 25mg의 [약물 이름]을 경구 투여함. 환자는 약물을 잘 복용하였으며 즉각적인 부작용은 나타나지 않음. 프로토콜에 따라 혈압 및 기타 활력징후를 모니터링할 예정.

연습 Scenario 1:
Intravenous medication administration

* Time: 10 minutes
* Setting: Surgical Ward
* Situation: A patient requires an intravenous dose of antibiotics for a chest infection, and the nurse must calculate and prepare the correct dosage based on the doctor's prescription.

✏ Example Scenario Description:

You are a nurse working on a Surgical ward. Mr. Kim, a patient, has been prescribed an intravenous antibiotic for a chest infection. The doctor's order specifies a 500mg dose, but the medication provided is in a 1g(1000mg) vial, requiring dosage calculation and dilution before administration.

Your task is to calculate the correct dosage, prepare the medication, administer it safely to the patient, and monitor their response. This scenario assesses your medication calculation skills, IV medication safety, and communication with patients.

Candidate Instructions:

1. Verify Medication Order and Check Patient Identity

- Cross-check the doctor's prescription and the medication provided. Follow the "7 Rights of Medication Administration"(Right Patient, Right Drug, Right Dose, Right Route, Right Purpose, Right Time, Right documentation). Use two identifiers(e.g., name and date of birth) to confirm patient identity.

What to say:

- "Good morning, Mr. Kim. My name is [Your Name], and I'm your nurse today. Can I confirm your name and date of birth? Thank you. I will be administering your antibiotic for chest infection treatment. Let me prepare the exact dosage for you."

2. Calculate Dosage and Prepare Dilution

- Based on the prescribed dose(500mg) and the provided medication(1g vial), prepare the dilution:
  - Dilute the vial as instructed(e.g., with 10mL of saline or sterile water).
  - Calculate the required volume:

(Thinking aloud):

- "The prescription is for 500mg, and the vial contains 1000mg. I need to draw up 5mL from the 10mL diluted solution to get the correct dose."

3. Explain the Procedure and Obtain Consent

➢ Explain the purpose of the medication and how it will be administered. Obtain verbal consent before proceeding.

What to say:
➢ "Mr. Kim, this antibiotic is to treat your chest infection. It will be administered intravenously for faster action. During the process, if you feel any discomfort or notice anything unusual, please let me know immediately. If you're okay with it, I will begin now."

4. Perform Hand Hygiene and Prepare the Medication

➢ Wash hands thoroughly and prepare the medication in an aseptic environment. Double-check the prepared dose and ensure proper equipment is ready for administration.

(While preparing):
➢ "I'm preparing your medication now. I've double-checked the dose and will ensure everything is correct before administration."

5. Administer the Medication and Monitor

➢ Administer the IV medication using the appropriate technique(e.g., IV push, IV piggyback). Monitor the patient for any adverse reactions during and after the administration.

What to say:
↳ "Mr. Kim, I'm starting the medication now. Please let me know if you feel any discomfort. I'll be monitoring you throughout the process."

6. Communicate and Document
↳ Document the dose administered, the time, and any observations. Communicate with the healthcare team if there are any adverse reactions or concerns.

What to say:
↳ "I've completed the medication administration and will record it in your chart. I'll continue monitoring you to ensure you're responding well."

<Common Antibiotics in New Zealand>

Intravenous Antibiotic	Oral Option	Oral Bioavailability
Amoxicillin	Amoxicillin 500 mg - 1 g TDS	72-93%
Amoxicillin clavulanate	Amoxicillin clavulanate 625 mg TDS	72-93%
Benzylpenicillin	Amoxicillin 500 mg - 1 g TDS	
Cefuroxime	Usually amoxicillin clavulanate 625 mg TDS	
Cephazolin	Cephalexin 1 g TDS	90%
Clindamycin	Clindamycin 450 mg - 600 mg TDS - QID	90%
Erythromycin	Erythromycin 400 mg QID	
Fluconazole	Same as intravenous dose	90%
Flucloxacillin	Flucloxacillin 1 g TDS	
Metronidazole	Metronidazole 400 mg BD (400 mg TDS for *C.difficile*)	80%

⑧ 의사소통 및 팀워크

Station Eight: Communication and teamwork

* Time: 10 minutes
* Setting: Inpatient Ward
* Situation: You are ending your shift and need to hand over the care of your patients to the incoming nurse.

⌲ Example Example Scenario Description:

You are a registered nurse finishing your shift on an inpatient ward. You are responsible for handing over the care of your assigned patients to the incoming nurse. This task involves using the ISBAR(Identity, Situation, Background, Assessment, Recommendation) format to ensure that critical information is clearly communicated, enabling a smooth transition of care. This scenario evaluates your ability to provide an effective handover and ensure continuity of care.

당신은 병동에서 근무하는간호사로써 근무를 마칠때, 자신에게 배정되었던 환자들의 케어를 다음 교대 근무 간호사에게 인계해야 합니다. ISBAR(Identity, Situation, Background, Assessment, Recommendation) 형식을 사용하여 중요한 정보를 명확하게 전달하고, 원활한 치료 전환을 보장해야 합니다. 이 시나리오는 효과적인 인계 과정을 제공하고 치료의 연속성을 보장하는 능력을 평가합니다.

Candidate Instructions:

1. Prepare a Structured Handover Using SBAR Format

Tasks:

- Organize the information for each patient into the ISBAR format:
  - **Identity:** your name, role, department(if they don't know you), Patient's name, age and location
  - **Situation:** Patient's diagnosis, and current issue.
  - **Background:** Relevant medical history and treatment received during your shift.
  - **Assessment:** Current condition, including vital signs, pain levels, physical assessment result, and any recent changes.
  - **Recommendation:** Next steps in care, such as pending tests, follow-up treatments, or potential concerns.

What to Say:

- "Let's start with Patient A. They are a 65-year-old male admitted for pneumonia. During my shift, their oxygen saturation dropped to 88%, requiring an increase in supplemental oxygen. Their vital signs

are now stable, but their respiratory rate is still slightly elevated."
- "I recommend monitoring their oxygen levels closely and administering the prescribed nebulizer treatment in the next hour."

> 먼저 환자 A부터 시작하겠습니다. 환자 A는 65세 남성으로 폐렴으로 입원하셨습니다. 제 근무 시간 동안 환자의 산소 포화도가 88%로 떨어져서 보조 산소를 증가시켜야 했습니다. 현재 vital sign은 안정적이나, 호흡수가 여전히 약간 상승해 있습니다. 환자의 산소 수준을 면밀히 모니터링하고, 다음 한 시간 내에 처방된 네뷸라이저 치료를 시행해야 될것으로 보입니다."

2. Clearly and Concisely Communicate Each Patient's Status

Tasks:
- Provide a brief summary of each patient, including their current status, ongoing treatments, and any notable changes during your shift.
- Use precise language to ensure the incoming nurse understands the key points.

> 각 환자에 대한 간략한 요약을 제공하며, 현재 상태, 진행 중인 치료 및 근무 시간 동안의 중요한 변화를 포함합니다.
> 정확한 언어를 사용하여 인계 받는 간호사가 주요 사항을 잘 이해할 수 있도록 합니다.

What to Say:
- "Patient B is a 72-year-old female recovering from hip surgery. She has been mobilized with assistance today and reports moderate pain at the incision site,

which is managed with analgesics. There's no sign of infection at the wound site."
- "Please ensure she continues to receive her pain medication as scheduled and assist her with mobilization as tolerated."

> 환자 B는 고관절 수술 후 회복 중인 72세 여성입니다. 오늘 도움을 받아 보행했으며, 절개 부위에 중등도의 통증을 호소했으나 진통제로 관리되고 있습니다. 상처 부위에 감염 징후는 없습니다."
> "진통제를 예정대로 계속 투여하고, 환자가 가능한 한 보행을 할수있도록 도와주세요."

3. Ensure the Incoming Nurse Understands Critical Information

Tasks:
- Allow time for the incoming nurse to ask questions and clarify any details.
- Confirm that they are aware of any urgent or time-sensitive tasks.

> 인계를 받는 간호사가 질문을 하고 세부 사항을 명확히 할 수 있는 시간을 제공하세요. 그 간호사가 긴급하거나 시간에 민감한 일에 대해 알고 있는지 확인하세요.

What to Say:
- "Do you have any questions about Patient C's medication changes? It's important that their anticoagulant is given on time due to their recent DVT."

↪ "If anything is unclear or if you need further information later, feel free to contact me before I leave."

> "Patient C의 약물 변경 사항에 대해 질문이 있나요? 최근 발생한 deep vein thrombosis(DVT) 때문에 항응고제가 제시간에 투여되는 것이 중요합니다."
> "혹시 불명확한 점이 있거나 추가 정보가 필요하면 제가 퇴근하기 전에 언제든지 연락하세요."

4. Document the Handover Accurately
Tasks:
↪ Record the details of the handover in the appropriate format or system, ensuring it is clear and complete.
↪ Include any significant updates, changes in treatment, and recommendations for the next shift.

> "적절한 형식이나 시스템에 따라 인수인계 세부사항을 기록하고, 명확하고 완전하게 작성합니다."
> "주요 업데이트, 치료 변경 사항, 그리고 다음 교대를 위한 권고사항을 포함합니다."

*What to Say:
↪ "I've documented all patient updates in the handover sheet. You'll find specific details about pending tasks and test results there as well."
↪ "Please review the documentation before starting your assessments to ensure nothing is missed."

> "환자 업데이트 내용을 모두 인수인계 기록지에 작성했습니다. 대기 중인 업무와 검사 결과에 대한 세부 사항도 거기에 있습니다."
> "환자 사정을 시작하기 전에 제 노트를 검토하여 누락된 사항이 없는지 확인해주세요."

연습 Scenario 1:

Interdisciplinary Team Meeting.

* Time: 15 minutes
* Setting: Inpatient Ward ? Conference Room
* Situation: You are participating in a multidisciplinary team meeting to discuss the care plan for a patient with multiple chronic conditions.

✎ Example Scenario Description:

You are a registered nurse participating in a multidisciplinary team meeting to review and plan the ongoing care of Mr. John Carter, a 68-year-old male patient with multiple chronic conditions, including congestive heart failure(CHF), type 2 diabetes, and chronic obstructive pulmonary disease(COPD). Mr. Carter was admitted two weeks ago due to worsening symptoms, including shortness of breath, lower extremity swelling, and unstable blood glucose levels. This scenario evaluates your ability to effectively contribute to a collaborative care plan while advocating for the patient's needs.

Candidate Instructions:

1. Present the Patient's Current Condition and Concerns

Tasks:
- Provide a concise summary of the patient's condition, progress, and any nursing concerns.
- Highlight key points, such as his recent symptoms, response to treatment, and any challenges with mobility, breathing, or self-care.

What to Say:
- "Mr. Carter has shown some improvement since admission, but there are still areas of concern. His lower extremity swelling has reduced with diuretic therapy, and his oxygen saturation is stable at 94% on 2L of oxygen. However, he continues to experience fatigue and reports difficulty walking short distances without becoming breathless."
- "We've also noticed fluctuations in his blood glucose levels despite adjustments to his insulin regimen. He expressed frustration about managing his diet and medications."

2. Listen Actively to Team Input

Tasks:
- Pay close attention to updates from the physician, physiotherapist, social worker, and other team members regarding their areas of expertise.

- Take notes on suggested interventions or changes to the care plan.

What to Say:
- "Thank you for sharing the plan to adjust his cardiac medications. I'll make sure we monitor for any side effects, such as hypotension or electrolyte imbalances."
- "I appreciate the physiotherapist's suggestion to introduce light exercises. I'll coordinate with Mr. Carter to encourage participation in breathing and mobility exercises."

3. Collaborate to Develop a Comprehensive Care Plan
Tasks:
- Contribute ideas from the nursing perspective, including patient education, symptom management, and monitoring strategies.
- Advocate for interventions that align with the patient's preferences and goals.

What to Say:
- "From a nursing perspective, I believe it's important to focus on educating Mr. Carter about managing his fluid intake and recognizing signs of fluid overload. We can also provide dietary counselling to help him better manage his diabetes."
- "He mentioned feeling overwhelmed by his

medications. Could we explore simplifying his regimen or involving a pharmacist for additional support?"

4. Advocate for the Patient's Needs and Preferences
Tasks:
- Ensure that the patient's voice is included in the care plan, particularly regarding his goals and concerns.
- Address barriers to adherence, such as low health literacy or limited mobility.

What to Say:
- "Mr. Carter has expressed that he values his independence and wants to avoid frequent hospitalizations. It's important we incorporate strategies to empower him, such as setting realistic goals for activity and self-care."
- "I'd recommend involving the social worker to assess his home environment for any barriers, like difficulty accessing healthy meals or challenges with transportation to follow-up appointments."

5. Summarize and Ensure Clear Communication
Tasks:
- Summarize the agreed-upon care plan and ensure each team member understands their role.
- Confirm that follow-up actions, such as scheduling tests or education sessions, are assigned.

What to Say:

- "To summarize, we'll focus on optimizing his medication regimen, providing ongoing education about fluid management and diet, and introducing a light exercise program. I'll also arrange for a follow-up with the social worker to address any home care needs."
- "If there's anything further to add or clarify, please let me know before we wrap up."

⑨ 간호계획 수립

Station nine: Planning nursing care

* Time: 10 minutes
* Setting: General Surgical ward
* Situation: A patient has just undergone abdominal surgery and requires comprehensive postoperative care.

✈ Example Example Scenario Description:

You are a registered nurse in a General surgical ward. Mrs. Sarah Thompson, a 58-year-old female patient, has just undergone an abdominal surgery(e.g., colectomy). You are tasked with assessing her condition, developing a postoperative care plan, and ensuring she and her family are well-informed and supported in the recovery process. This scenario evaluates your ability to assess a patient's postoperative condition and create a comprehensive care plan to ensure proper recovery.

당신은 일반외과 병동 간호사입니다. 58세 여성 환자인 사라 톰슨(Mrs. Sarah Thompson)은 복부 수술(예: 결장 절제술)을 방금 마친 상태입니다. 당신은 그녀의 상태를 평가하고, 수술 후 간호 계획을 수립하며, 그녀와 그녀의 가족이 회복 과정에서 충분한 정보를 제공받고 지원을 받을 수 있도록 해야 합니다. 이 시나리오는 환자의 수술 후 상태를 평가하고 적절한 회복을 보장하기 위한 포괄적인 간호 계획을 수립할 수 있는 능력을 평가합니다.

Candidate Instructions:

1. Conduct a Thorough Assessment of the Postoperative Condition

- Assess vital signs(blood pressure, heart rate, respiratory rate, temperature) and pain level.
- Examine the surgical incision for signs of infection(e.g., redness, swelling, drainage).
- Evaluate the patient's comfort and mobility level, noting any difficulty with movement or breathing.

활력 징후(혈압, 심박수, 호흡수, 체온)와 통증 수준을 평가하세요.
수술 절개 부위를 검사하여 감염 징후(예: 발적, 부기, 배액)가 있는지 확인하세요.
환자의 편안함과 보행 수준을 평가하며, 움직임이나 호흡에 어려움이 있는지 확인하세요.

What to say:

- "Good morning, Mrs. Thompson. I'm here to check on you after your surgery. I'll start by taking your vital signs to ensure you're recovering well."
- "I'll also examine your incision site to make sure there are no signs of infection. Are you feeling any pain or discomfort right now?"

> "안녕하세요, 톰슨 씨. 수술 후 몸상태가 어떠신지 확인하려합니다. 먼저 활력 징후를 측정하여 회복 상태가 좋은지 확인하겠습니다."
> "절개 부위에 감염 징후가 없는지 확인하려 하는데요, 현재 통증이나 불편함이 있으신가요?"

2. Develop a Care Plan

↝ Plan for effective pain management, considering both pharmacological(e.g., analgesics) and non-pharmacological methods(e.g., positioning, relaxation).

↝ Identify potential complications such as infection or deep vein thrombosis(DVT) and plan for early intervention.

↝ Plan for early ambulation to promote circulation and prevent complications like pneumonia and DVT.

> 약물 치료(예: 진통제)와 비약물 치료(예: 자세 조정, 이완 요법)를 포함한 효과적인 통증 관리를 계획합니다.
> 감염이나 Deep Vein Thrombosis(DVT)과 같은 잠재적 합병증을 인지하고 조기 중재를 계획합니다.
> 순환을 촉진하고 폐렴 및 DVT와 같은 합병증을 예방하기 위해 조기 보행을 계획합니다.

What to say:

↝ "We'll work together to manage your pain and make sure you're as comfortable as possible. I'll be administering medication to help manage any discomfort, and we'll also use positioning to minimize pain."

- "It's also important for you to start moving around as soon as we can to avoid potential complications. I'll assist you with gentle ambulation to help you regain strength and improve circulation."

"통증을 관리하고 환자분이 가능한 한 편안하게 지낼 수 있도록 저희 의료진은 함께 노력할 것입니다. 불편함을 줄이기 위해 약물을 투여할 것이며, 통증을 최소화하기 위해 자세를 조정하는 부분도 고려할 것입니다."
"잠재적 합병증을 예방하기 위해 가능한 빨리 움직이기 시작하는 것도 중요합니다. 제가 에너지와 혈액 순환을 개선할 수 있도록 보행을 도와 드리겠습니다."

3. Plan for Nutritional Support and Fluid Balance

- Plan for the initiation of a postoperative diet, starting with clear liquids and advancing to solid foods as tolerated.
- Ensure adequate fluid intake to prevent dehydration and promote wound healing.

"수술 후 식이 계획을 시작합니다. 먼저 맑은 액체부터 시작하고, 환자분께서 잘 소화를 시키시면 점차 고형식으로 진행합니다."
"탈수를 예방하고 상처 치유를 촉진하기 위해 적절한 수분 섭취를 보장합니다."

What to say:

- "We'll start you on clear liquids today to make sure your stomach is ready for food after surgery. Once you're able to tolerate that, we can move on to solid foods."
- "It's important to stay hydrated to support your recovery, so I'll monitor your fluid intake throughout the day."

> "오늘은 맑은 액체로 식사를 시작하겠습니다. 이는 수술 후 위가 음식을 받을 준비가 되었는지 확인하기 위한 것입니다. 이를 잘 소화하시면 고형식으로 진행할 수 있습니다."
>
> "회복을 돕기 위해 수분 섭취를 유지하는 것이 중요합니다. 하루 동안 수분 섭취량을 모니터링하겠습니다."

4. Communicate the Care Plan to the Patient and Family

- Clearly explain the care plan to the patient, ensuring they understand the postoperative instructions and the importance of follow-up care.
- Discuss potential complications and how to recognize signs of infection, bleeding, or other concerns.
- Provide the family with an understanding of the care plan and how they can support the patient's recovery at home.

> 환자에게 간호 계획을 명확히 설명하고, 퇴원 후 지침과 추후 관리의 중요성을 이해하도록 돕습니다. 발생할 수 있는 합병증 및 감염, 출혈 또는 기타 문제의 징후를 인식하는 방법에 대해 논의합니다. 가족에게 간호 계획에 대해 설명하고, 가정에서 환자의 회복을 지원할 수 있는 방법을 안내합니다.

What to say to the patient:

- "You'll need to follow some important instructions after you leave the hospital. This includes caring for your incision site, managing pain, and knowing when to seek medical help."
- "If you notice any changes, such as increased redness, swelling, or drainage from your incision, or

if you develop a fever, please let us know right away."

"퇴원 후에는 몇 가지 중요한 지침을 따라야 합니다. 여기에는 절개 부위 관리, 통증 조절, 그리고 의료 도움이 필요할 때를 아는 것이 포함됩니다."
"만약 절개 부위에 발적, 부기, 또는 분비물이 증가하거나, 발열이 발생하면 즉시 저희에게 알려주세요."

What to say to the family:

↷ "It's important that we work together to support Mrs. Thompson's recovery. She may need assistance with walking and managing her pain at home. I will provide you with specific instructions to ensure a smooth transition from hospital to home."

토마슨 씨의 회복을 돕기 위해 함께 노력하는 것이 중요합니다. 환자분은 집에서 보행부분과 통증 관리에 대한 지원이 필요할 수 있습니다. 병원에서 집으로 원활히 전환할 수 있도록 구체적인 지침을 제공해 드리겠습니다.

연습 Scenario 1:
Chronic Disease Management

* Time: 10 minutes
* Setting: Discharge Planning Area
* Situation: A patient with chronic heart failure is being discharged home and requires a comprehensive chronic disease management plan.

🖉 Example Scenario Description:

You are a registered nurse preparing a 72-year-old male patient, Mr. John Williams, for discharge after an extended hospitalization due to chronic heart failure exacerbation. Mr. Williams is ready to go home, but he requires ongoing management to prevent future complications. Your task is to assess his current health status, develop a care plan to manage his chronic heart failure and ensure that he and his family are fully prepared to manage his condition at home. This scenario evaluates your ability to provide patient education and create a sustainable care plan that will optimize the patient's health outcomes.

✍ Candidate Instructions:

1. Perform a Comprehensive Assessment of the Patient's Current Health Status

- Review the patient's medical history and current medications, ensuring that he understands his prescribed medications and their side effects.
- Assess the patient's dietary habits, including fluid intake and sodium consumption, which are critical in managing heart failure.
- Evaluate the patient's physical activity level and determine his readiness to resume or adjust his exercise routine, in line with his heart failure status.
- Review any recent lab results(e.g., electrolytes, kidney function) and vital signs, and note any trends that may impact his discharge plan.

What to say:

- "Mr. Williams, I'll go over your medications one more time to make sure you understand how to take them, and I'll check if there are any concerns. We also need to talk about your diet, particularly how to manage sodium intake and fluid balance."
- "How are you feeling physically right now? Are you comfortable with any changes in your activity level? It's important to balance rest and movement to avoid unnecessary strain on your heart."

2. Develop a Care Plan for Chronic Heart Failure Management

- Include medication management, ensuring the patient is clear on the purpose of each medication(e.g., diuretics, ACE inhibitors) and the importance of adherence.
- Recommend dietary modifications, particularly reduced sodium intake and proper fluid management, to avoid exacerbations of heart failure.
- Plan for daily weight monitoring to detect fluid retention early and assess the need for adjustments in diuretic therapy.

What to say:

- "To manage your heart failure at home, you'll need to weigh yourself every day at the same time, ideally in the morning, to keep track of any fluid retention. If your weight increases by more than 2-3 pounds over 2-3 days, you'll need to contact the doctor."
- "I'll go over your medications once again, and I'll make sure you understand the proper doses and timing. We need to stick to your prescribed regimen for the best results."
- "Your diet will be essential in preventing your heart failure from getting worse. I'll provide you with guidelines for a low-sodium diet and help you understand which foods to avoid."

3. Plan for Patient Education on Recognizing Heart Failure Exacerbation Symptoms

- Educate the patient on recognizing early warning signs of a heart failure exacerbation, such as increased shortness of breath, swelling in the legs or abdomen, weight gain, or fatigue.
- Emphasize the importance of seeking medical help promptly if any of these symptoms worsen or if new symptoms appear.
* Provide written materials or resources that reinforce these key concepts for reference at home.

What to say:

- "It's very important that you know what signs to look out for at home. If you experience sudden shortness of breath, swelling in your legs, or if you feel more tired than usual, it's time to contact your healthcare provider."
- "I'll provide you with a pamphlet that outlines these symptoms, so you'll have a reference to guide you in case you're unsure about whether or not to seek help."

4. Arrange for Follow-up Appointments and Community Resources

- Schedule follow-up appointments with the cardiologist or primary care physician to monitor the patient's heart failure status.

↪ Provide information on community resources, such as heart failure support groups, nutrition counseling, or home health services, to ensure ongoing support.

What to say:
↪ "I've scheduled your follow-up appointment with your cardiologist for next week. It's important to keep that appointment so we can check your progress and make any necessary adjustments."
↪ "There are also community resources available, including support groups for patients with heart failure. These groups can help you connect with others who are managing similar challenges."
↪ "If you ever feel overwhelmed with managing your condition at home, don't hesitate to call the clinic, or we can refer you to home health services for additional support."

⑩ 위급한 상태의 환자 관리

Station Ten: Managing the deteriorating patient

---

* Time: 10 minutes
* Setting: Acute medical assessment Unit
* Situation: A patient with a history of COPD is experiencing acute respiratory distress.

✒ Example Example Scenario Description:

You are a registered nurse caring for Mr. Thomas Clark, a 72-year-old patient with chronic obstructive pulmonary disease(COPD), who is presenting with acute respiratory distress. Mr. Clark is exhibiting signs of increased work of breathing, laboured breathing, and a decrease in oxygen saturation. The patient's family is also visibly concerned about his condition. Your task is to perform a rapid assessment, provide appropriate interventions, and communicate effectively with the healthcare team to ensure optimal patient care.

당신은 만성 폐쇄성 폐질환(COPD)을 앓고 있는 72세 환자, 토마스 클락(Mr. Thomas Clark)을 돌보는 간호사입니다. 현재 클락 씨는 급성 호흡 곤란 증상을 보이고 있으며, 호흡 일량 증가, 호흡 곤란, 그리고 산소 포화도 감소와 같은 징후를 나타내고 있습니다. 환자의 가족 또한 그의 상태에 대해 눈에 띄게 걱정하고 있습니다. 당신의 과제는 신속한 평가를 수행하고 적절한 중재를 제공하며, 최적의 환자 치료를 보장하기 위해 의료팀과 효과적으로 소통하는 것입니다.

Candidate Instructions:

1. Perform a Rapid Assessment

- Assess the patient's respiratory status by checking vital signs, including respiratory rate, heart rate, and oxygen saturation levels.

환자의 호흡 상태를 사정하기 위해 호흡수, 심박수, 산소 포화도 등 활력 징후를 확인합니다.

- Listen to the patient's lung sounds to identify any abnormal findings, such as wheezing, crackles, or diminished breath sounds.

환자의 폐음을 청진하여 천명음, 수포음, 또는 호흡음 감소와 같은 이상 소견이 있는지 확인합니다.

- Observe the use of accessory muscles of respiration(e.g., neck muscles, intercostal retractions) and assess the patient's level of distress.

호흡 보조 근육(예: 목 근육, 갈비뼈 사이의 근육 사용)의 사용을 관찰하고 환자의 고통정도를 평가합니다.

- Evaluate the patient's ability to speak, noting any difficulty in forming sentences, which may indicate worsening respiratory failure.

> 환자의 말하는 능력을 평가하고 대화시 문장을 형성하는 데 어려움을 겪는지 확인합니다. 이는 호흡 부전이 악화되고 있음을 나타낼 수 있습니다.

What to say:

- "Mr. Clark, I'm going to check your breathing now. I need to know if you're feeling any tightness or difficulty when you breathe."
- "I'll listen to your lungs to see if we can find out what's causing your breathing issues."
- "We need to check your oxygen levels, so I'm going to place a small clip on your finger to measure it."

> "클락씨, 환자분의 호흡 상태를 지금 확인하겠습니다. 숨을 쉴 때 답답하거나 어려움이 있는지 말씀해주세요."
> "폐음을 청진하여 호흡 문제의 원인을 확인해 보겠습니다."
> "산소 포화도를 확인해야 하니, 손가락에 작은 클립을 붙여 측정하겠습니다."

2. Administer Oxygen Therapy and Prepare for Intubation

- Administer supplemental oxygen as prescribed, starting with a nasal cannula or non-rebreather mask, depending on the severity of the oxygen saturation drop.
- If the patient's condition does not improve, prepare for the possibility of intubation, ensuring the necessary

equipment is ready and the respiratory team is alerted."
- Maintain a calm and reassuring presence with the patient to help alleviate anxiety, which can exacerbate breathing difficulties.

> 산소 포화도가 떨어진 정도에 따라 비강 캐뉼라나 비재호흡 마스크를 사용하여 처방된 산소를 공급합니다. 환자의 상태가 호전되지 않으면, 기관 삽관 가능성에 대비하여 필요한 장비를 준비하고 호흡기 팀에 알립니다. 환자의 불안을 완화하기 위해 차분하고 안심을 주는 태도를 유지합니다. 불안은 호흡 곤란을 악화시킬 수 있습니다.

What to say:
- "I'm going to give you some oxygen to help you breathe easier, Mr. Clark. This should help improve your oxygen levels."
- "If your breathing doesn't get better, we may need to assist you more with breathing support. Let's see how the oxygen helps first."
- "I know this is difficult, but I'll be right here with you to support you through this."

> "클락 씨, 숨을 좀 더 쉽게 쉴 수 있도록 산소를 공급해드리겠습니다. 이 산소가 산소 수치를 개선하는 데 도움이 될 것입니다."
> "만약 숨쉬기가 나아지지 않으면, 더 많은 호흡 지원이 필요할 수도 있습니다. 우선 산소가 얼마나 도움이 되는지 지켜보겠습니다."
> "이 상황이 어렵다는 것을 알고 있습니다만, 제가 도와드릴 테니 걱정하지 마세요."

3. Monitor Vital Signs and Respiratory Status
- Continuously monitor the patient's oxygen saturation, respiratory rate, and heart rate.
- Watch for signs of worsening distress, such as

increased use of accessory muscles, cyanosis, or a significant drop in oxygen saturation.
- Keep track of any changes in the patient's condition and document these promptly.

> 환자의 산소 포화도, 호흡수, 심박수를 지속적으로 모니터링합니다. 보조 근육 사용 증가, 청색증 또는 산소 포화도 급격한 감소와 같은 악화 징후를 주의 깊게 관찰합니다. 환자의 상태에 변화가 있을 경우 이를 신속하게 기록하고 문서화합니다.

What to say:
- "I'm going to check your oxygen level again in a few minutes to make sure we're getting the right amount of oxygen to help you."
- "I'll also be checking your heart rate and breathing closely, so I can make sure we're moving in the right direction."

> "몇 분 후에 산소 포화도를 다시 확인해서 적절한 산소가 잘 공급되고 있는지 확인하겠습니다."
> "심박수와 호흡수를 면밀히 확인하여, 상태가 잘 나아지고 있는지 확인하도록 하겠습니다."

4. Notify the Physician and Collaborate on Management
- Notify the physician immediately about the patient's deteriorating condition and the need for further intervention.
- Collaborate with the healthcare team to adjust the treatment plan, which may include more aggressive

interventions, such as mechanical ventilation or administration of bronchodilators.
- ✒ Ensure that the physician is aware of any changes in the patient's condition, including respiratory status and vital signs.

> 환자의 상태가 악화되고 추가적인 처치가 필요함을 즉시 의사에게 알립니다. 의료 팀과 협력하여 치료 계획을 조정하며, 이는 기계적 환기나 기관지 확장제 투여와 같은 보다 적극적인 처치를 포함할 수 있습니다. 환자의 호흡 상태와 활력징후를 포함한 상태 변화를 의사에게 확실히 전달합니다.

What to say to the physician:
- ✒ "Dr. Lee, I have a 72-year-old patient with a history of COPD who is showing signs of acute respiratory distress. His oxygen saturation is dropping, and he's using accessory muscles to breathe. I've started oxygen therapy, but he's not improving."
- ✒ "We may need to consider more advanced interventions like intubation if his condition worsens."

> "Dr. Lee, COPD 병력이 있는 72세 환자가 급성 호흡 곤란 증상을 보이고 있습니다. 산소 포화도가 떨어지고 있으며, 호흡을 위해 보조 근육을 사용하고 있습니다. 산소 요법을 시작했지만 상태가 호전되지 않고 있습니다."
> "환자의 상태가 악화될 경우, 기도삽관과 같은 처치를 고려해야 할 수도 있습니다."

5. Document Findings, Interventions, and Communications
- ✒ Accurately document the initial assessment, including the patient's respiratory status, vital signs, and any interventions provided, such as oxygen therapy.

- Record any communications with the physician or respiratory team regarding the patient's care.
- Ensure that the documentation is clear, detailed, and timely, providing a complete record of the patient's condition and the care provided.

> 환자의 초기 평가 내용을 정확히 기록합니다. 여기에는 환자의 호흡 상태, 활력 징후, 산소 요법과 같은 처치가 포함됩니다. 환자의 치료와 관련하여 의사나 호흡 치료 팀과 나눈 모든 의사소통 내용을 기록합니다. 문서는 명확하고 상세하며 시기적절해야 하며, 환자의 상태와 제공된 치료에 대한 기록을 제공합니다.

What to say:
- "I'm going to note everything we've done so far in your chart to ensure we have a full record of your care today. This will help keep track of your progress."

> "환자분, 오늘 치료 과정을 완전하게 남기기 위해 지금까지 했던 모든 것을 차트에 기록하겠습니다. 이것은 당신의 상태가 어떻게 나아지고 있는지 추적하는 데 도움이 될 것입니다."

연습 Scenario 1:
Acute Stroke

* Time: 10 minutes
* Setting: Emergency Department
* Situation: A 72-year-old patient presents with sudden-onset facial drooping, slurred speech, and weakness on one side of the body, indicating a possible stroke.

✈ Example Scenario Description:

You are a nurse in the emergency department and Mr. David Taylor, a 72-year-old patient, has presented with signs of acute stroke. He has sudden facial drooping, difficulty speaking, and weakness in his right arm and leg. Time is of the essence, and you must act quickly to assess the situation and prepare for potential thrombolytic therapy or other interventions.

Candidate Instructions:

1. Perform a Rapid Assessment

- Assess the patient's level of consciousness using the Glasgow Coma Scale(GCS) and check for signs of a stroke using the FAST acronym(Face drooping, Arm weakness, Speech difficulties, Time to call for help).
- Check vital signs and measure oxygen saturation, as low oxygen levels may worsen stroke outcomes.

What to say:

- "Mr. Taylor, can you smile for me? I'm going to check your arm strength. Please raise both arms for me."
- "We need to act quickly, so I'll need to check your vital signs and start preparing for the doctor."

2. Notify the Physician and Prepare for Thrombolysis

- Notify the physician immediately about the symptoms and urgency of the situation.
- Start preparing the patient for possible thrombolytic therapy, which requires timely administration within a certain window.

What to say to the physician:

- "Dr. Roberts, we have a 72-year-old male presenting with right-sided weakness, facial drooping, and slurred speech, consistent with an acute stroke. I've started the initial assessment and am preparing for thrombolytic therapy."

3. Monitor Vital Signs and Oxygenation

- Continuously monitor the patient's blood pressure, heart rate, and oxygen saturation.
- Ensure that the patient's oxygen levels are within an acceptable range and provide oxygen if necessary to improve perfusion.

What to say:

- "I'm going to check your oxygen levels now to make sure you're breathing comfortably, Mr. Taylor."
- "I'll keep monitoring your vitals as we get ready for the next steps in your care."

4. Prepare for Potential Transfer to Stroke Unit

- Ensure the patient is stable for transport and prepare to transfer them to a specialized stroke unit or neuro ICU for further care.

What to say:

- "We're going to get you to a special unit that focuses on treating strokes, Mr. Taylor. I'll be with you every step of the way."

5. Document Findings and Actions

- Document all observations, assessments, interventions, and communications related to the stroke. Ensure that all actions taken are clearly noted in the patient's chart.

What to say:
- "I'll be noting everything in your chart so that the team knows exactly what's been done to help you so far."

포널스 참고문헌

장수향. (2018). **뉴질랜드 간호사 되기**. 포널스.

김미연. (2019). **국제간호사 길라잡이**. 포널스.

손정화. (2020). **국제간호사 호주편**. 포널스.

송원경. (2021). **국제간호사 두바이편**. 포널스.

정해빛나. (2021). **국제간호사 미국편**. 포널스.

김소미. (2022). **국제간호사 사우디, 조지아편**. 포널스.

간호사적응연구소. (2023). **병원적응 의학용어**. 포널스.

간호사적응연구소. (2023). **국제간호사 병원영어 Vol1 - 말하기 편**. 포널스.

간호사적응연구소. (2023). **국제간호사 병원영어 Vol2 - 간호상황 편**. 포널스.

백소연. (2024). **미국간호사 밥줄영어 vol 1권**. 포널스.

백소연. (2024). **미국간호사 밥줄영어 vol 2권**. 포널스.

간호사타임즈. (2024). **태어난 김에 국제간호사**. 포널스.

윤보혜. (2024). **국제간호사 호주(탈임상)편**. 포널스.

이지원. (2024). **미국 부자 간호사 가난한 간호사**. 포널스.

강은진. (2025). **선넘는 간호사 - 호주간호사로 선넘다**. 포널스.

간호사연구소. (2025). **간호알고리즘 PRO-A1 호흡기내과**. 포널스.

간호사연구소. (2025). **간호알고리즘 PRO-A2 심장내과**. 포널스.

간호사연구소. (2025). **간호알고리즘 PRO-A3 혈액종양내과**. 포널스.

간호사연구소. (2025). **간호알고리즘 PRO-A4 소화기내과/간담췌내과**. 포널스.

간호사연구소. (2025). **간호알고리즘 PRO-A5 신장내과**. 포널스.

간호사연구소. (2025). **간호알고리즘 PRO-A6 일반외과/정형외과**. 포널스.

간호사연구소. (2025). **간호알고리즘 PRO-A7 신경외과**. 포널스.